What Can I Give You?

∽

Mary Mahony

Redding Press
Belmont, Massachusetts

Second printing 2000

Susan A. Pasternack, Editor
Holly McGovern, Designer
Bang Printing, Brainerd, Minnesota

Medical photographs on pages 155–157 by James W. Koepfler, Children's Hospital, Boston
Photographs on pages 158 and back cover ©Joe Demb, Belmont, Massachusetts

"The Gift" by Gregory A. Denman from *When You've Made It Your Own* used with the kind permission of Heinemann, a division of Greenwood Publishing Group, Portsmouth, NH, 1988.

For background on the origins of Boston Floating Hospital and Children's Hospital, Boston, we are indebted to the following sources: *Doctor and Teacher, Hospital Chief: Dr. Samuel Proger and the New England Medical Center* by Herbert Black, The Globe Pequot Press, Copyright ©1982 by New England Medical Center, Inc.; *The Children's Hospital of Boston: "Built Better Than They Knew,"* by Clement A. Smith, M.D., Little Brown and Company, Copyright ©1983 by Clement Smith, M.D.; and *Children's World,* Spring 1994, Office of Public Affairs, Children's Hospital.

Library of Congress Catalog Card Number: 97-91901
ISBN 0-9658879-0-1

To my most precious gifts, my children,
Breen, Colin, and Erin

Contents

∞

PROLOGUE

⁓

This is a very personal account of one family's struggle with congenital scoliosis. In medical terms, congenital scoliosis refers to a disorder of the spine that can lead to a very severe deformity. Although the word congenital literally means "born with," this problem is not inherited in the genetic sense. Rather, something happens to the developing embryo at a very early stage, perhaps even before a woman realizes that she is pregnant. All degrees of severity are possible with this disorder, from a deformity of the trunk that is obvious at birth to a hidden defect that may take years to make its presence felt. In its most severe form, progress can be very rapid, necessitating early and repeated treatment to maintain some semblance of control.

The spinal abnormality can be very complex. Scoliosis implies a curvature of the spine in the side-to-side direction, but this can be combined with deformities in the forward (kyphosis) or backward (lordosis) direction, in any degree.

Associated spinal abnormalities include a spike of bone that pierces the spinal canal (diastematomyelia), resulting in damage to the spinal cord which can lead to varying degrees of paralysis of the limbs if not detected early and treated properly. In addition, the spinal cord can be tethered at the lower end, causing a progressive problem with leg function. Frequently there is a deformity of the chest cage with ribs either missing or fused together. Increasing spinal curvature can also lead to a chest deformity becoming progressively severe.

Other organ systems can be involved and once the diagnosis of congenital scoliosis is established, a search must be made for co-existing problems in both the cardiac and genitourinary systems, as these develop at the same time as the spine and can be affected by the same unknown cause.

Deformities of the spine itself are a result of faulty programming in the very complex process of development of the separate bones (vertebrae) that make up the spinal column. In some instances, some of the growth centers

7

on one side of the spine can be joined together instead of separated. This tethers the involved side, leaving the other side to continue to grow, resulting in a progressive curvature — a condition known as a unilateral bar (a bar to one side), which can produce the most severe form of distortion and usually requires surgical attention as early as the first year of life. Since the area involved with the bar has no potential for growth in length, the choice is between a short, relatively straight spine or a short, crooked one. Experience has shown that if only the back surface of the spine has been fused, the involved portion of the front of the spine may continue to grow, causing secondary deformity. Early fusion naturally results in a shorter spine, but that shortened spine is due to the original problem and not to the fusion.

A less severe form of the disorder is caused by a vertebra that has formed only on one side (hemivertebra). If detected early and subjected to surgery if progressive deformity occurs, the effects can be minimized. The majority of cases of hemivertebrae are not progressive and only require close observation. If early progression is detected, then an operation on the front and back of the spine can either arrest or correct the deformity.

It must be obvious then that children with congenital scoliosis must be carefully monitored by examination and periodic X rays to see if the deformity is worsening. If this is confirmed, there is no place for a "let's wait and see" attitude or any attempt to correct the problem with a brace. However reluctant a parent may be to consider surgery in a very young child, it is the only answer.

When the child reaches teenage with an uncorrected curve or one which has begun to progress during the rapid growth phase, the operation can still be performed, but it is obviously more complex and carries additional risks, particularly to the spinal cord. The operation may have to involve removing a wedge of the spine and will certainly involve the placing of metal rods to correct the curve as much as can be done safely and maintain the correction until the spinal fusion is solid.

The effect of a severe spinal deformity on a child can be devastating and cause great heartache for both the child and the parents. The impact can be minimized by early, effective surgical treatment. Moreover, not all congenital scoliosis requires treatment, an assessment that can only be made by someone familiar with complex problems of the spine. The surgeon who specializes in spinal deformities in children will make that determination based on X rays and other studies. Although the advice given may be hard to take, it is not as hard as the consequences of a neglected severe spinal deformity.

The difficulties experienced by this family and so carefully chronicled here are worthwhile reading by parents of children who face similar problems.

John E. Hall, M.D., Senior Associate, Children's Hospital, Boston
Professor of Orthopaedic Surgery, Harvard Medical School

ACKNOWLEDGMENTS

O ur journey with Erin may not be unlike one which you have taken with your child. Ours was a much easier trip than that of some families. There are children all over the world who are born every day with birth defects or who become chronically ill. These children are an inspiration to all of us who can come out of ourselves and realize that our day-to-day issues are nothing compared to what these children face. And it is thanks to the doctors at medical facilities such as the Floating Hospital, Children's Hospital in Boston, the University of Kansas Medical Center, and many other fabulous medical facilities that we can hope for a healthier future, if not for our own child, for those who come after. A special thanks to Dr. Lester Abelman; Dr. Max Ramenofsky; Dr. Michael Goldberg; Dr. R. Michael Scott; my uncle, Dr. Walter Boehm, who died in August of 1994; Dr. Len Cerrulo; Dr. Marc Asher; and Dr. John Hall, and the many other supportive people who added and continue to add to the richness of Erin's life. Most of all, Kevin and I would like to thank Erin's brothers, Breen and Colin. Their loving support could be a whole other book.

INTRODUCTION
What Is a Child?

⟨∞⟩

Bringing a child into this world is a far more serious undertaking than many of us realize. It is an honor, a privilege. Bringing a normal child into this world is about the greatest gift a parent can ever bestow. When that child isn't normal, no matter how mild the problem, it opens the gates to a completely different experience. Suddenly, you lose control over many aspects of parenting. It is as if someone simply yanked it all out of your hands and, almost immediately, you begin to find ways to get that control back. You look to the world of the specialist, embarking on an exhausting journey, the scope of which you are too numb and too naive to imagine.

As I reflect on my own experience as a parent-to-be, for the most part I felt both responsible and prepared. As with all new ventures, you don't really know what it's going to be like until you get there. Certainly, I never expected perfection, but as I look back, I'm not sure I fully expected anything less than normal. Not perfect, but normal. Today, some twenty-five-plus years since I gave birth to my first child, I realize what a distorted view I had. "Normal" has many different connotations, but I was far too inexperienced to realize this at the time. If someone asked me today what a normal child is, I'd probably laugh that such a ridiculous question was even being posed.

⟨∞⟩

Our story begins a quarter century ago. My husband, Kevin, and I were not unlike many other young people who had landed in Boston for graduate school, fallen in love with the area, and decided to give it a go permanently. Kevin hailed from New York, a city boy at heart, while I came from a small town in western Connecticut. We eventually settled in Belmont, Massachusetts, a small bedroom community near Boston where we seemed to have found the best of both worlds — the proximity to a large and bustling city and a yard full of trees. In time we became the parents of two boys and were ready to welcome our third, and perhaps last, child.

CHAPTER ONE
A Premonition

⌒

Pregnancy for me was always a difficult time. I am small and on each occasion felt as if I had given birth to future fullbacks. I will never forget the look of disbelief on the face of the medical resident who delivered my oldest son, Breen, who weighed in at nine pounds six ounces and measured a little more than twenty-two inches long. I left the hospital a mere ninety-eight pounds.

After mothering two very active boys, Breen and Colin, for five and a half years, I decided to try one last time, hoping for someone who might sport a dress on occasion or perhaps a barrette or two. I assumed that I'd end up with "My Three Sons," but a tiny part of me wanted very much to deliver the female vintage. However it turned out, I was thrilled to be a mother once again.

During the final weeks of carrying this third one, I was very uneasy. The baby was restless and the pregnancy uncomfortable. The activity inside my small body was really bringing the rafters down and I worried that something was wrong. When "labor day" finally arrived, I had very mixed feelings but was pretty sure I would be buying more airplane underwear. So on January 31, 1978, when this gorgeous, chubby female, soon to be named Erin Margaret Mahony, came out weighing in at eight pounds ten ounces, I felt that once again someone was truly watching over me.

Erin was an extremely attractive little baby with lovely features: beautiful peach-like skin and a tiny rosebud mouth. That wonderful closeness that I felt from the very first time I held her would be what carried us through the times ahead.

Like her brothers before her, Erin needed a soy-based formula as she had difficulty fully digesting those made from milk. In the hospital she seemed a bit cranky, but then again, so was I. We both had a lot of adjusting to do. The first day home she fussed for nine hours. I suppose you'd call her colicky, but in retrospect, I believe that there were other things going on in her tiny body as well. Fortunately, my mother had come to my rescue, excited about seeing her first new granddaughter in sixteen years. Indeed, it was she who saved the day and helped cement my relationship with Erin from the very beginning. In the midst of my frustration, my mother somehow succeeded in calming us both down while answering the door and the phone and dealing with everything else that arose.

The other great advantage I had at the beginning (and I'm probably the only one to say this) was the arrival in New England of "the blizzard of '78," which provided me with a lot of snow to entertain my boys, no school schedules to adhere to, a husband who could not possibly find transportation to his office, and a mother who was forced to stay two weeks longer than she had planned. Best of all, having just given birth, I couldn't possibly shovel.

By the time my mother left and the troops were back in school, Erin and I were the best of friends. During these early days my doorbell rang constantly and I often felt that I had accomplished some great feat by having a baby girl. The visitors came for a variety of reasons. The friends who had two children wanted to see what sort of chaos three brought. Those with only one kid looked at me in awe and offered their deepest sympathy. The families with all boys came to see if girls really felt different, and the ones with no children went home and bought dogs. Whatever their reasons for coming, I enjoyed the company and always had a pot of coffee and lots of funny stories.

With a six-month leave of absence from my job in special education I welcomed their visits but knew that I would soon need to resume my busy life. So when Erin was a month old I slowly began to return to some of my activities. I have always been an extremely energetic person, able to complement motherhood with other interests. In addition to teaching Saturday-morning special-education classes for my church, I led workshops in this area for the Archdiocese of Boston. I was also involved in a variety of local organizations.

As the days passed, Erin seemed to be adjusting well to her new surroundings and, with the exception of some minor difficulty in digesting her food, everything was fine. But as summer drew near she fell victim to a rather constant series of ear infections and at one point she even developed strep throat. Fortunately, we had a wonderful pediatrician, Dr. Lester Abelman, who dealt with Erin's various maladies with both competence and compassion.

As Erin passed her three-month birthday, I began to feel unsettled. Despite my many outside interests, I made the decision not to return to my part-time job when my leave was up and monitored my other activities as well. Although Erin's checkups were fine, her vomiting problem seemed to be increasing and her ear afflictions were growing more complicated. And yet, her spirit and ever-present smile were always in place.

I also noticed that Erin showed little interest in crawling, although that did not really concern me at the time. Colin, my second child, did not move off his haunches until he was eight and a half months old and tired of his older brother taking his trucks away. I assumed my daughter was simply another late bloomer.

In April of 1978, when Erin was a little more than three months old, I discovered a small growth inside her right check. Although relatively unconcerned, Dr. Abelman and I decided that we'd both feel better if a pediatric surgeon had a look. In no time we were off to Boston's Floating Hospital.

The Floating, which traced its beginnings to the late nineteenth century and Boston harbor, was now the pediatric unit of the New England Medical Center, a well-known hospital complex located downtown on the fringe of what was once known as Boston's "Combat Zone" area. Leaving the small provincial office of our pediatrician for a large urban medical center was a rather intimidating experience. I remember clearly my very first impression as we entered surgeon Max Ramenofsky's waiting area. The seriousness and degrees of illness I observed there were the extreme rather than the norm. I knew that children's woes came in all shapes and sizes, but seeing them all together in one room was truly overwhelming.

Dr. Ramenofsky was a wonderful pediatric surgeon who had come highly recommended by Dr. Abelman. After reading Erin's brief history, he checked her over thoroughly, assured me that the tiny growth in her mouth was probably benign, but set a surgery date of June 2 just to be safe. Since Erin would be admitted as an outpatient, we'd only be there part of the day. I left Dr. Ramenofsky's feeling relieved and a bit silly for being so concerned. But I had my work cut out for me keeping Erin healthy in the ensuing weeks. Summer is pretty reliable when it comes to weather, but with Erin there was never any guarantee.

The morning of the scheduled surgery we awoke early. While dressing Erin, I noticed a drizzle from one of her nostrils. I couldn't believe my eyes! Oh darn, we're never going to make it today. And although we proceeded with our preparations, it was clear that anesthesia would be out of the question.

When Dr. Ramenofsky came in to discuss a new date, Erin started showing signs of hunger. She had not eaten in several hours in preparation for the surgery. "Go ahead and feed her," he encouraged. So, while he and I talked, Erin enjoyed her first meal in several hours; less than ten minutes later she had created a rather striking wall mural. If the sight didn't turn your stomach, the smell did.

Prior to this rather vivid experience I had not thought of discussing Erin's digestive condition since it seemed to have peaks and valleys and she was gaining weight steadily. I was soon to discover that gastroesophageal reflux, an inability for the food to pass through the reflux valve into the stomach, was one of Dr. Ramenofsky's specialties as well as one of Erin's problems. His concern was most apparent and he proceeded to discuss her digestive system at great length as well as her ear infections.

Following this review, Erin and I proceeded upstairs to the radiology department for an "upper G.I." series of X rays to see what was going on in Erin's tummy. I soon began to notice how well my defense system functioned. My light and humorous side began to surface and I appeared to be the mother who could handle anything. But I can still remember how lonely I felt inside. While awaiting Erin's return, I set my sights on a mural of Big Bird from *Sesame Street* and counted how many brush strokes it took to give him feathers. Truly, at this point, I was the featherhead!

On our return Dr. Ramenofsky studied the test results, gave me a pamphlet on gastroesophageal reflux, and explained why the vomiting had not subsided. To avoid surgery he wanted Erin strapped onto her crib mattress at a 60° angle for sleep in an attempt to force the food to flow downward into her stomach. The alternative was a "Bobby-Mac" carseat in which she'd sleep sitting up, at the same 60° angle. If all else failed, the final resort would be surgery. But Dr. Ramenofsky reminded me several times that he had found great success with the less radical approaches. We also decided to proceed with placing tubes in Erin's ears since her repeated infections showed no signs of improving.

By the time Erin and I left the Floating Hospital that June day she had an appointment with Dr. Ramenofsky for removal of her mouth cyst (papilloma) and another with the ear, nose, and throat specialist for placement of ear tubes, as well as complete instructions regarding eating and sleeping routines. Our plate seemed pretty full, or so I thought.

❧❦

Back home, propping up Erin's mattress and holding her at a 60° angle was a real challenge. After trying many arrangements, I discovered a way of securing an elastic belt around her back and tummy and placing pillows at the bottom of the bed to secure her position. With all these adaptations, she finally seemed able to rest in one place. A real triumph! I used to tell my friends that I was the mother of a nine-month-old baby who slept "ready for takeoff!" And as with everything else in her life, Erin adjusted beautifully and Dr. Ramenofsky was right; the food did stay down.

The day for Erin's mouth surgery finally arrived, and it felt good to wheel her off to the operating room. While I awaited the completion of the procedure, it suddenly dawned on me how dramatically Erin's life had changed and in such a short time. Then I caught myself in mid-thought as I sat there watching the other children in the room with far more serious problems than Erin's. Their mothers looked so tired and yet, somehow, they were able to share some very genuine smiles. I admired them for the warmth they showered not just on their own little ones, but on the others in the room as well.

I was rescued from my reverie when a nurse announced that Erin was all set. A drink of Kool-Aid and she was ready for action. The cyst was indeed benign so we were able to go home without delay. I left the hospital feeling very positive and relieved that Erin's ordeal was finally over.

⌒⌒

Following surgery, life felt a little bit more settled. The winter holidays, my favorite time of the year, would soon be upon us and Erin seemed to be doing great. Breen and Colin had learned to deal with the extra time I spent with their little sister, especially after meals, and life appeared pretty normal.

But with Erin sleeping at an angle, my daily schedule was very different from what it would have been otherwise. She woke up at least once each night in need of readjusting, understandably so: sleeping on a runway, half in the air, was not easy. But for me, these were the quiet moments when I could get a warm, half-conscious hug, the bonus when any of our children needed me in the middle of the night. I'm a light sleeper and have never required huge amounts of rest, so the interruptions were very manageable.

Unfortunately for Erin, she was still not able to spend much time playing on all fours with her brothers since the activity of crawling seemed to disturb her reflux problem. At times I felt very envious of those mothers whose little ones were showing signs of walking. Then I'd remind myself that I had raised two lazy boys who had taken their time, too. Erin just sort of crept along enjoying each day.

The holidays came and went with the usual chaos that one expects from three children and lots of company. Always fairly well organized, I proceeded with things at my usual pace. Even before Erin I had always looked like Phyllis Diller during Christmas vacation week!

By early January Erin's vomiting had completely subsided and she was crawling around like a little mouse. Dr. Ramenofsky gave his okay to leave the runway and come in for a landing. I was overjoyed. Finally, Erin could sleep like the rest of the tots in the world. I had some concerns over her recurring ear problems, although the tubes in her ear canals seemed to help and the infections were coming with less frequency. So while Erin started to enjoy the life of a normal twelve-month-old, I slowly began to resume some of my old activities on a more regular basis. Life seemed to be going along very well and I was feeling very, very fortunate.

∞∞

It was soon February of 1979. Erin's first birthday was behind us and I was feeling quite upbeat. The boys were enjoying school and the rush and craziness of the holidays had passed. Erin was crawling around more and more and she was holding her food down very nicely.

Along the way I had acquired the habit of feeling around Erin's mouth to make sure there were no additional growths. While I probed, she would watch me with this very disgusted look on her face as if to say, "Feel around your own mouth." Her facial expressions were always a dead giveaway, even at a mere thirteen months, and as I think about it, I wouldn't want anyone stretching my cheeks and feeling around my mouth either.

Then one night in early February I discovered what I hoped I wouldn't: another growth. All my worst fears returned. I was especially alarmed when it appeared to be in the same location as the first. I was extremely relieved when Dr. Abelman was able to confirm that this was not the case, yet we were both a bit baffled. He immediately arranged for me to return to Dr. Ramenofsky. I had a three-week wait.

The time before the visit seemed to pass by normally for everyone but me. I tried to be positive but, in truth, I was really more nervous than before. I hated the thought of Erin having anesthesia again, however minor the surgical procedure. She was getting bigger and becoming much more aware of the wider world. She had recently suffered through a terrible cold and I felt that the poor little kid had no respite from the world of doctors and medicine. But she could have cared less. Her life seemed to revolve around two little stuffed ducks. While not always in the best of shape, the ducks were her mascots, her best friends. They followed her everywhere, sharing their own mutual admiration society.

CHAPTER TWO

Premonition to Reality

⌘

On March 22, 1979, our appointment day arrived. I awoke early to get the boys off to school and to prepare Erin and her ducks for yet another trip to the Floating Hospital. I knew Erin would not be overjoyed once we arrived there so I prepared a variety of snacks, healthy ones, not fat pills. At the age of fourteen months she found food very dear to her heart, especially an unsolicited treat.

By the time we arrived at Dr. Ramenofsky's office at nine o'clock, it was already wall-to-wall with kids and nervous parents. The area was very cheery and alive with the activity of many busy, but smiling, members of the medical staff. The bustle of the atmosphere was a marvelous distraction and my anxiousness was lost in trying to entertain Erin and the handful of little ones that always gather around a playful mom.

I was relieved when Dr. Ramenofsky's nurse signaled and led us to a back examining room. Erin was once again beginning another heavy cold, but I figured that in examining her Dr. Ramenofsky would pick up on this and rescue us from having to see yet another doctor. And I hoped he could prescribe something for her cough.

Although I had only met with Dr. Ramenofsky three or four times, I had a lot of confidence in his ability to relate to both Erin and me. He was very personable and always enjoyed a wonderful one-sided dialogue with Erin. As he began his examination, she was less than cooperative. But he was quick and very thorough. Once again he believed that the growth was not serious, but was baffled as to why she had another.

My fears were allayed, and I asked if he could also check out her cough; her congestion and discomfort were quite apparent. As I went about undressing Erin, Dr. Ramenofsky looked over her file. I observed that he took careful note of her back and appeared to do a double-take. I began to feel very uneasy. Behind the dressing table where Erin was sitting stood a full-length mirror. He continued to stare at her back, moving again and again between the mirror and the table. As he did this, we talked about Erin's inability to stand up or hold on very well. It was clear to me that he was one very concerned doctor and I became one very concerned mother.

As Dr. Ramenofsky proceeded to go over every inch of Erin's back, he motioned for his nurse and then left to make a phone call, explaining that he wanted the counsel of another physician. I could feel a huge lump taking up residence in my throat and I knew we were in trouble. I wanted someone to tell me everything was just fine, but I knew that was not going to happen.

After a short wait, the other doctor arrived. It was very apparent that he had come directly from the operating room. He was quite rushed and yet there was no doubt in my mind that he knew exactly what he was looking for and whatever that was, Dr. Ramenofsky had felt it was serious enough to get him down from surgery. My greatest concern was not what he was seeking, but whether or not he would find it.

∞∞

The doctor who came to examine Erin that March day was orthopedic surgeon Michael Goldberg and today he is a dear friend. As I think back to that very first meeting, it always puts a smile on my face. He came down to the examination room in a very untidy-looking doctor's coat. You could tell he had rushed because his hair looked like he had just taken a drier to it and, to beat all, his tie was on backwards and, on a very chilly March day, he wore no socks. In spite of it all, he had such a thoroughness about him that everything else seemed unimportant. And, in fact, all the other was unimportant.

Dr. Goldberg was both honest and positive and yet I could see he had some serious concerns about the little body before him. He briefly tried to explain that the apparent curvature he and Dr. Ramenofsky were seeing in Erin's spine could be quite serious and he outlined two possibilities, each a type of congenital scoliosis: one demanded very careful monitoring and constant follow-up while the other would require all that and possibly major surgery. He spoke of the latter very briefly and assured me that this was rare and that I shouldn't concern myself with this until more tests were done. He then arranged for Erin to have several X rays before we left that day. As I stuttered through twenty questions, he assured me that he would call at six o'clock sharp that evening with the results.

I couldn't remember a time in my life when I felt such fear of the unknown. As I stood there dressing Erin in silence, Dr. Ramenofsky and his nurse knew exactly what I was thinking without asking. They were outstanding and yet they knew, even better than I, that there was nothing anyone could say. They wanted me to call my husband, but I explained that he was en route to Atlanta on business and wouldn't be back for three days. I just wanted to get Erin ready, give her a big hug, and move on.

As I proceeded to dress Erin, I felt as if I was in a scary movie that I wished would end so that I could leave the theater and go back to reality. But in my heart I knew it was all real and that it would probably be frightening for a long, long time. The term "congenital scoliosis" had me so distracted that I almost forgot what I was supposed to be doing. Thoughts of a recent school committee meeting I had attended in my town preoccupied me. A woman named Bunny Gowen, founder of the National Scoliosis Foundation, had come to petition for scoliosis screening in our schools. During the session she had shared some rather worrisome facts, but what really scared me when I recalled the talk was learning that a particular kind of scoliosis, "idiopathic," could be more easily corrected, unlike the other types, which were often caused by different, more serious birth defects. It seemed so bizarre that this was the only school committee meeting I had attended in almost a year and that scoliosis had been the evening's topic.

<hr />

I soon realized the effect my silence was having on Erin. This patient little munchkin was looking up at me as if to say, "Can't I be included in this conversation?" Because we were an unscheduled appointment, we had a long wait in radiology and passed the time with some other young patients. When the X-ray technician finally arrived, Erin was less than cooperative about saying good-bye to the kids. Thank God the technicians noticed her toy ducks and took them along. Bedraggled as they appeared, the birds sure came in handy and Erin could not have found a more dependable set of friends.

As I look back, I remember so clearly how isolated I felt. I was so overwhelmed that it took all of my remaining energy to even think of how I would arrange for my sons Breen and Colin, who hadn't a clue that my day was any different from any other. As I was rearranging the boys' schedule over the phone, I didn't realize how this one short visit was already reshaping our lives, especially Erin's.

When Erin reappeared, her face looked as if she was covered with the latest in skin rashes: all those tears had really left their mark. The technician felt awful. In time Erin would learn that being X-rayed would become the determining factor in many of the health-care decisions yet to be made. This time it was just another hospital experience.

Finally, it was time to go. Driving home to pick up the boys I put my mind on "fast forward," wondering what kind of impact all this would have on our family. I knew that change is never easy for children, most especially when it has something to do with health.

As I pulled up to Colin's nursery school, the friend whom I had called as a backup was getting out of her car. I could feel the tears welling up so I very briefly explained our day without going into too much detail. I had all I could do to just try to be myself, let alone talk to anyone. I was so relieved that Breen was at a friend's house. The thought of no more explanations put my mind at ease. I simply wanted to be home. I was feeling kind of weird and different, as if I was starting on a journey that someone was forcing me to take. There was no time to reorganize and begin packing; I was already on my way.

After I unloaded everyone, I had a few short moments to myself. I thought about some of the other children Erin and I had seen at the Floating whose burdens were far greater than ours. Erin was an alert, bright, healthy little girl who was possibly facing a life with a disability. I thought I should feel relieved that it wasn't anything worse.

In retrospect, I now realize what a difficult time this was for our boys. Normally when Breen and Colin came home, I would sit down and ask how their day went. My agenda was now very different. The distraction of Erin's situation and Kevin's being away made me very preoccupied. Fortunately, Colin had a personality that you'd like to bottle and market. My distraction didn't alter his program one bit, because to him, life was a smile and a matchbox car.

Breen, then a first-grader, took everything very seriously and found it difficult to share his feelings or to have someone share theirs with him. The least bit of change in his daily pattern was disturbing. He was a serious child, so for him this would be very, very major. My thoughts went from Erin, to Colin, to Breen, and then to Kevin, because he was the farthest away.

With all this on my mind I decided to get the kids organized and put Erin in for her nap. I no sooner got her settled than the phone rang. It was Kevin calling from the Atlanta airport to see how Erin and I had fared. As I recall this conversation, which I have replayed in my mind at least a thousand times, I realize that it probably would have been better and much easier on Kevin if I had only addressed the growth in Erin's mouth. But I didn't choose that course. Telling someone long distance that his child may have a birth defect or serious illness is not easy. No matter how you say it, it's rather upsetting, a moment that you remember for the rest of your life.

⚬⚬⚬

At about six that evening Dr. Goldberg called, just as he had promised. I remember well where I was standing. He had read Erin's X rays and things did not look good, but he could not be sure without a myelogram, a test in which they drain the spinal fluid and inject a dye into the spinal column to provide a complete "picture" of the area.

According to Dr. Goldberg, Erin's X ray revealed a progressive curve of 27–30°, a very substantial angle for a child her age. He wanted to make a date for further tests as soon as possible and asked if I had any questions. It was at that point that I said it would be helpful if both Kevin and I came in to see him. Dr. Goldberg was wonderful and suggested that we bring Erin in together on the following Tuesday during Kevin's lunch hour. So we firmed up the date, March 27, 1979, at noon, and said good-bye.

As I hung up the phone I felt reassured that this doctor, whom I hardly knew, was at least able to recognize our needs as well as Erin's. Physicians need to remember to consider the dynamics of the whole family as a unit, not simply the person they are treating. To me it's like learning spelling vocabulary. If you don't learn how the word is used in a sentence and how it relates to the other elements, you really haven't learned much about that word at all. Dr. Goldberg knew his lessons well and understood that this medical "package" involved much more than just Erin.

⚬⚬⚬

When I put the boys to bed that night, I was feeling some sadness about their day. I remember sitting down on the bottom of their bunk beds and explaining that Erin had a problem. We talked about her not walking yet nor standing for very long. Then I explained that even though her tummy was better and she wasn't getting sick anymore, maybe there was something else we needed to find out. Although I knew they were listening, they looked as if they could have cared less. A conversation about trucks would have been much more appealing.

As I think back on that night, I now understand that what I was feeling was guilt. Why had I not seen the curve? How could I have missed it when I could see it so clearly in the doctor's office? I was also concerned that Erin was in pain. She was far too little and too happy to provide any clues. As I sat there putting myself through the third degree, I could finally piece together so many of Erin's problems, going all the way back to my difficult pregnancy. I wandered back upstairs and peeked in her room. There she was, fast asleep, looking so perfect, so healthy. I thought to myself, What can I give you Erin? How can I make this all go away and make you better? I'm sure many parents of children with birth defects ask themselves this same question. Although I had done all the obvious things, I felt that I should have been giving something more, but I couldn't, for the life of me, figure out what.

Kevin returned from Atlanta and found discussion extremely difficult. We were both devastated by the news but experiencing it in different ways. I had had a few more days to process the information. I was able to accept the possibility of the diagnosis being correct and yet Kevin was struggling and being very closed about the whole issue. I had also already begun to reorganize my life and prepare for all that might await us.

People's reactions to the news were amazing and I was finding out who my friends were and where their priorities lay, both family and others. Fortunately, all through my life, I have been blessed with many good and wonderful friends. At this time they were more important than ever; their ongoing support was a gold mine. No matter how much I needed, they were always there, and at times, I felt as if our friendships had become a one-way street. But they never put up a detour.

ೞ ೞ

Tuesday, March 27, did not come soon enough. Kevin's extremely brusque manner during the meeting with Dr. Goldberg was an immediate indication that all his defenses were up and that he was in full control, probably on "overdrive." He always made me uneasy when he was like this, but we all have our own way of dealing with difficult situations or perhaps not dealing. It's those who refuse to accept the situation on any level that I worry about. This is not something to ignore.

Dr. Goldberg was very friendly and extremely thorough, making us feel very much at ease. This was our first formal meeting and he acknowledged that our initial contact was unplanned and had occurred under unusual circumstances. He explained how very rushed he had been and how he had needed to go back to whatever he was doing prior to Dr. Ramenofsky's call. This session had a much better feel to it. Kevin listened attentively and processed the medical facts with great ease. Dr. Goldberg suggested that we get a second opinion to alleviate any doubts we might have. He gave us the names of two other doctors at Children's Hospital in Boston and urged us to move quickly. He explained that more tests were crucial in the event that other unforeseen problems might exist.

At this point the hardest thing for me to understand was why Erin didn't seem to make much of an attempt to walk. In the back of my mind I was pretty much convinced that whatever was wrong with her had affected that development. But I needed to focus myself on the day-to-day and as Dr. Goldberg had said to us, "Do what is best for Erin." His presentation was very direct. His concern was that she be followed and that we have the necessary tests done. He held back nothing. Most important, he talked about our needing good medical insurance because the process would be costly. He really put it all out on the table. Some doctors present so poorly that you feel as if you've been hit by a Mack truck while others offer maudlin sop aimed only at assuaging what should be real concern. Dr. Goldberg's explanation was neither.

At this stage, Kevin seemed to be far more optimistic than I. As the mother and caretaker, I was the one who was feeling the changes each day. I often envied that Kevin had a daily change of scenery; for me, that was virtually impossible. I knew that I would have to set the tone so that the boys could go on with their schedules, Kevin would have his needs filled, and Erin would receive good care and support. Could I possibly grow more arms and legs? Would I have the time and the opportunity to give the boys the emotional support they would need? Would I be able to be there for them and for Erin as well?

⌒⌒

My first task was to get a second opinion. That was easier said than done but I must highlight the importance of the second opinion and sometimes even a third, if the first two are drastically different approaches. There were no appointments available for several months with the doctors that had been suggested. I was not at all prepared for this. Doesn't the whole world stop for you when you find out your child is ill? After many frustrating phone calls, I decided to go with Dr. Seymour Zimbler, another orthopedic surgeon at the Floating, and to have Erin's X rays sent to my Uncle Walt, a neurosurgeon who lived in Tennessee. I knew my uncle would be able to consult with one of his orthopedists down there and get word back to me. I was fortunate to have such a resource.

Our appointment with Dr. Zimbler was scheduled for mid-April. Unable to find a slot for us during the day and aware of the urgency of the situation, he agreed to see us in the evening. I was impressed by his willingness to accommodate our needs. During the month preceding our visit, it looked to me as if Erin's curve was increasing. I was very anxious to hear what he had to say about all this. Like all mothers, I kept hoping it was my imagination.

Dr. Zimbler had a formal way about him. He was very pleasant but fired away with many questions in an effort to get to know Erin's history. Upon looking at her X rays and examining her, he felt it hard to believe that I had not seen some indication of her back problem. I explained to him that once, in the bathtub, she appeared a bit lopsided but I thought it was the angle at which I was looking as well as her chubbiness. With two active little boys at my side everything was rush, rush, rush. Also, Erin's reflux problem had limited her activity. I focused on that so my attention was on her front, not her back. In addition, she had missed her most recent pediatric checkup due to a flu. Maybe I should have seen the curve, but the point was, I hadn't. It was a question that I turned over and over in my mind on a daily basis. In time, I learned not to be so hard on myself.

Dr. Zimbler suggested that Erin's inability to walk might be due to a problem on her left side. There was a discernible difference between her left and right feet and calves. He urged us to admit her to the hospital as soon as possible for a week of tests. He gave us no guarantees in regard to her walking someday but merely said, "Let's do first things first."

Before leaving Dr. Zimbler, Kevin had organized his mind clearly enough to ask some key questions. He inquired as to how long Erin would be immobile if surgery was necessary. The projected time was three to six months, but that could soon change after the severity of Erin's damage was ascertained. It was clear to me that we were about to embark on a whole new life. What no one prepared me for was the variation in coping skills that I was about to see in those around me. The silence in the car on the way home was deafening. We had a long road to travel.

On the positive side, I felt fortunate that the doctors were on the right track and that Erin was a mere fifteen months old. I was optimistic that just maybe we were in the right place at the right time. Erin was also very strong. For such a little lady, her coping skills were impressive. I felt that she'd probably deal with this one, too, so long as everyone else was able to do their part.

CHAPTER THREE
Diagnosis Confirmed

The next day I began communicating with Dr. Goldberg's office, urging them to admit Erin as soon as there was an opening. I was anxious to know the extent of her damage. I felt that I had a big cloud over my head and wondered if it would sprinkle or rain bullets.

Dr. Goldberg's secretary, Rose, kept the channels of communication open. Spring was a busy time and I was only one of many parents looking for a bed for their child. When I came out of my cocoon I realized that the delay had nothing to do with the season of the year; illness and inpatient numbers varied like the weather.

Rose was wonderful to us and even came through with the private room I requested. Kevin took the week off from work so I could live at the hospital. Looking back, I was very fortunate that I was free to be able to do that. Many parents did not have that option because they both had to work. You just can't imagine how hard it was for some of them.

Finally, on May 14, Erin entered the Floating. At this point I was ready for the diagnosis and welcomed the opportunity to find out what else lurked in that small body. It was a time of such uncertainty. Our first destination was for blood work. Being a poor sport about such things myself fully prepared me for Erin's reaction, but I had already decided to take a supportive stand. In isolation, a blood test is very minor, but for Erin it was just the beginning of a long, difficult journey. My job was to help her cope with it all. Sometimes, as the years wore on, I'd go to bed feeling like a real "creep" because I had to serve as Erin's conscience for all that she would eventually have to do for her back. When the day finally arrived for her to serve as her own counsel, I felt a great sense of relief; but still, I worried. For some parents, that day never comes: the situation forces their children to be dependent for life.

From the labs, we headed up to Erin's room. When we arrived, I noticed that all the patients in this area seemed to be hooked up to or in some kind of orthopedic gear. I had landed on a whole new planet! At first, it shocked me to think that so many children had to go through so much just to get started in life. The nurses sensed my mood and made a special effort to accommodate us.

Within minutes after we arrived, a third-year medical student came in with pen and paper in hand. As he proceeded to examine Erin, she commenced a fit of screaming that broke the sound barrier. The student and I ignored it in hopes that she might calm down. In a very loud voice, so as to be heard over Erin's screaming, I attempted to answer an endless list of questions. If you are ever in our situation, remember to bring the medical archives with you. All the questions wore me down. But there were good reasons for it all and I appreciated the thoroughness — at least, I did in the end.

Dr. Skenck, Dr. Goldberg's assistant resident at the time, took good care of us that first night. I'm sure my look of concern and desperation was a sure clue to what was passing through my mind. When you move into a hospital room for a week, all the parents of the children in the other rooms drop in to see what your child has and you, in turn, ask the same of them. It serves as a somewhat necessary form of support. It bonds you. You develop a spirit of caring for one another that stays with you throughout your life. When I look through Erin's photo album of that week, I remember the cast of characters as if it were yesterday.

Since Erin and I had a private room as I had requested, my cot was right next to her crib. There was barely space for the nurses to walk between us. I definitely think that I was "overbonding" that week.

The next morning, after being seen by a fanfare of very serious M.D.'s, Erin went off for her IVP test (intravenous pyelogram) to see how her kidneys were functioning. The IVP indicated an anatomical abnormality that is very common in patients with congenital scoliosis. Erin's ureter, the tube that goes from the kidney to the bladder, was double. Fortunately, everything was functioning fine in spite of this and everyone felt that she had passed the test with flying colors. I was later told that some children who have Erin's birth defects also suffer from renal failure.

After a good nap, Erin shoved off for an hour of tomograms, X rays that focus on a specific area while excluding surrounding structures. I requested that they let me in so that Erin would be more cooperative. At first radiology hesitated, but they could see that she was not a happy camper and decided that perhaps, if I could calm her down, the tests, which involved a lot of turning and twisting of the patient, could be done without having to medicate her. So whenever Erin began her fit of crying, I threatened to leave. I felt awful, but it worked, and she was absolutely terrific. Even the radiologist commented on how composed she had been. Seeing your child being twisted and turned is a bit of a shock at first. I had to keep telling myself that it would really help Erin if we could just get on with all this. In reality, the tests were pretty harmless and it was all the clutter of the situation that made it seem stressful and a bit scary.

The radiologist read Erin's tomograms and as I look back, that was the beginning of our bad news. He found her curve to be approximately 38°. On March 22, the day she had first been seen by Dr. Goldberg, it was 27°, so I became alarmed that in less than two months the curvature had increased so dramatically.

The next morning Erin was scheduled for the myelogram. The anesthesia team paid me a visit the evening before and explained that they would drain out the spinal fluid from Erin's spine and then inject a dye. The doctor noted there was always a risk involved with such a test and in order for them to do this procedure, he needed my signature. So I signed and off he went.

Dr. Goldberg arrived promptly at seven the next morning for rounds. They had already given Erin her "sleepy" shot so I was able to give him my undivided attention. His concern was most apparent. Not only was Erin's curve extensive but her spine appeared rigid in some areas which meant, in layman's terms, that perhaps it would not be easily manipulated. He had also decided to keep Erin an extra day for another test, an electromyogram, to see if there was any bladder damage. I assumed that meant that if there was, Erin might never be toilet trained.

Although Dr. Goldberg was both thorough and attentive to my inquisition, I felt the need for some family support so I decided, once again, to call my uncle in Tennessee. I needed reassurance and support that went far beyond what Dr. Goldberg could give. Erin was not his only patient. As always, my uncle was very reassuring as well as cautious. He never really answered my question as to where this was all leading. How could he? He was in Tennessee and we were in Boston. But he assured me that I was in the very best of hands, which I already knew.

Early the next morning, Dr. Barger, another of Dr. Goldberg's residents, came in to say that there was a definite obstruction found on Erin's myelogram and then put me on hold until Dr. Goldberg arrived. The wait was very difficult. Dr. Goldberg soon popped his head in and with him came more bad news. But his presentation was so good that although I was very worried, I felt a great deal of support. He reported that a neurosurgeon, Dr. R. Michael Scott, would arrive soon and that Dr. Scott could best explain to me what the obstruction was and how we needed to address it.

⌒⌒

Dr. Scott's arrival left me with a sense of both relief and anxiety: relief that I would finally get a detailed answer and anxiety that I might not like what I was going to hear. His presentation was very serious, but incredibly warm and loving to Erin. It was clear that he enjoyed children and was also very keenly aware of the plight of the parent at a time like this. I could see that he was moved by Erin's pretty face as were many of the people who had met her throughout this ordeal.

Dr. Scott explained that Erin had a double bone spur (diastematomyelia) or piece of bone piercing the spinal canal, lodged between two thoracic vertebrae, T-9 and T-10. I could hardly pronounce the word, let alone grasp how it got there. He sensed my confusion and went on to elaborate that it was rare but that he had seen and operated on others before Erin. This particular bone spur had caused and continued to cause serious neurological problems for Erin on her left side, which explained the weakness I saw in her left leg and the difference between her left and right feet and calves. No wonder she didn't walk or stand up for more than a few seconds. He pointed out that there was also nerve damage that would have to be addressed. Things were not looking good and I suddenly felt the need for a back transplant for Erin.

Erin's complete diagnosis was as follows: Butterfly vertebrae at T-10, hemivertebrae on the right at T-11, fused rib T-10 to T-12: absent pedicle on the left T-11, and an unsegmented bar T-10 to T-12. In addition, there was a diastematomyelia at T-9, T-10.

Dr. Scott went on to say that in light of the extent of what had been found, surgery needed to be done as soon as there was an available slot. He outlined the two-part operation: first, he would perform the necessary neurosurgery to remove the bone spur and then, during the same procedure, Dr. Goldberg would proceed and do some fusing of Erin's hemivertebrae. Dr. Scott explained that due to the thickness of Erin's bone spur, he might not be able to remove all of its anterior extent. He felt optimistic about the outcome of surgery, however.

After Dr. Scott left, I just sat there for a few minutes, absolutely numb. Poor Erin didn't know what was going on and I suddenly realized that she was there, staring at me, probably wondering if I had lost my ability to speak. I quickly gathered myself together as best I could and picked her up.

After a few big hugs I read a story and then gave her those infamous duckies and told her I had to phone her dad. How I dreaded that call. Kevin was not at all prepared for the extent of Erin's damage and I could tell he was not processing everything I was saying. It wasn't your typical telephone call and yet there was no way to minimize the information. He had taken the week off to handle the boys and, at that point, I'm sure he was feeling pretty frazzled. I still maintain that the job at home can be a lot more exhausting than one outside. The unpredictability of a normal day with children can be a challenge. Finally, I suggested to Kevin that he gather the boys together and come to the hospital. I really missed them, as did Erin, and I think we all needed to be together.

In the meantime, I again called Uncle Walt in Tennessee and shared with him as best I could what Dr. Scott had told me. I did a little more checking around in the Boston area and found out that Dr. Scott was a top-notch neurosurgeon and extremely well respected far beyond the region. We needed to put our trust in the hands of both doctors and do everything possible to make this a good experience not only for Erin, but for everyone.

The next morning, Erin had a urodynamics test to ascertain any bladder damage. I won't explain in detail how the test is done but it was quite uncomfortable for her and her young age seemed to have an effect on the doctor who was performing it. Sensing my concern and exhaustion, he allowed me to observe the camera and watch the actual functioning of Erin's bladder. I felt quite relieved when he announced that all was well. At least we had won that round. I had also received a lesson in physiology that I would never forget. I was mellowed by the whole experience and once again reminded myself of how much we take for granted.

The next morning was discharge day. Our week of tests was finally coming to a close and another chapter in our lives had ended. I was overwhelmed by the thought of what the next would offer.

ᗧᗡ

On May 18, 1979, we arrived home. It was great to get hugs from the boys and finally see my own kitchen again. Although it felt good to be home, it didn't take long for me to realize that life was feeling more complicated. Our smiles were a bit artificial and there was a level of anxiety and worry that we were still trying to process. Unfortunately, I thought that it was my job to help everyone cope. At the time, I could have saved an enormous amount of energy and worry if I hadn't tried to carry it all myself.

The time had come to share the news of Erin's test results with family members. Telling my mother was probably the hardest for me. She had watched me struggle through the pregnancy and knew how much I loved kids. Prior to Erin's birth, my mother had suffered a serious stroke. Her recovery was incredible but not surprising to any of us. She was a very strong woman but equally sensitive. I hated the thought of giving her something to worry about. She is a true lover of children and she is as patient as she is caring. I am very lucky to have her.

As the days passed I spent my time reading everything I could possibly get my hands on related to congenital scoliosis. There was really very little information and what was available was either very basic or oriented to the physician. As a result, I was left feeling totally in the dark. I also did a little asking around about Drs. Goldberg and Scott, although I felt very confident with our choice or rather their choice of us.

With time I was getting more comfortable with Erin's coming surgery and I talked about it freely when people asked. The perspectives of the physician and the parent are not always as different as one might think. It was clear to me that my concern was shared by both of Erin's physicians. Although Dr. Scott was encouraging, he had this one facial expression that was less relaxed than his usual presentation, and over the years, I would watch for it whenever we discussed Erin.

Each day brought new emotions and it was really my sense of humor that got me through the tough times. I used to dig down and pull it out just to get through. Comic relief has always been my best defense. I seemed to find my greatest amusement in the reactions of other people. Some were extremely supportive; others were not. I learned to excuse them all and felt that some were in worse shape than Erin would ever be. My quick wit and honest mouth abruptly halted some pretty strange responses and at the same time, rescued what I guess I would very loosely call a "friendship." I knew Erin would survive but I was a bit worried about some of the others.

It also became very clear who my real friends were. I was touched by their generous support. They found a million excuses to stop by or call and even though, at the time, I thought being alone would be better, I needed them more than words can ever say. I came to understand the value of friendship on a whole new level.

❦

The ensuing weeks got rougher for Erin. She developed an ear abscess and I was pretty anxious about keeping her healthy for her surgery. Through it all, Dr. Abelman really earned a gold star. Surgery slots were hard to come by and I was nervous Erin might not make it in on her designated day. That would not have been the end of the world but at the time, I probably would not have agreed.

Balancing my time with the boys and getting them comfortable with all this was a bit of a stretch. I dearly loved them and their traditional little spats and active lives certainly served as a distraction to all the other stuff that was in my head. I tucked them in each night and gave them an update and made sure I let them know that I would still have plenty of time for them. Mostly, they sat there giving me their "cripe" look, wondering who was going to sleep on the top bunk and who would get the bottom. It was pretty wild, but I knew that in spite of it all, they were listening.

As we moved closer to surgery, I had to curtail some of Breen's activities. I felt terrible, but it involved so much carpooling. I never realized how much time I spent in the car until I sat down trying to figure out what the boys could continue to do and what was not at all realistic. As I sit here writing, thinking back, I realize the many changes the boys' lives went through in such a short time. Kevin was working and I was always tending to Erin without the benefit of an extended family around to bail us out. It amazes me how well everyone survived. When I think of the families who have it so much worse than we did! These people became my role models and taught me things that you could never find in a book.

Our last adventure before Erin's surgery was a trip to one of our town's more famous portrait studios, Ben Franklin's. Did I say portrait studio? Really, Ben Franklin's was about as eclectic as Belmont got in those days. They had a big sign in the window advertising a portrait special. The boys refused to wait in line so the next day I just took Erin. I'm sure she wasn't thrilled, but she complied, and I was happy to get one last photo of her "plaster-less."

CHAPTER FOUR

The Longest Day … and After

O n June 18, 1979, Erin and I set off for the Floating once again. I was fortunate that Erin's godmother, Rose, who lived in New York and had known Kevin and his mother for years, had agreed to come up and stay with the boys. Rose had only one child, a daughter named Ria, who was developmentally delayed. Ria was born at a time when there was little acceptance of mental retardation and so Rose had spent much of her life seeking the best care for her daughter. Rose was a fantastic mother and friend and for these qualities we had selected her to be Erin's godmother. It had seemed an automatic choice.

It was hard to send the boys off to school that morning knowing I wouldn't be the same mom for a while. And that's okay so long as you share your insight with those around. Preoccupation changes the dynamics of anything pretty quickly and I was already aware things would be a bit different. The boys needed a clue, too.

At the hospital Erin and I were first sent off to the pediatric clinic for her physical to make sure she was a good candidate for surgery. We had a marvelous resident who was most impressed with Erin and taken with her pretty face. Erin seemed to feel comfortable and before long we were thanking the resident and on our way. As we were departing, I heard the doctor calling to us. I turned to see what I had forgotten. "Good luck," she said. "This place is wonderful, so don't worry." Those extra words of support meant a great deal.

The lab work was next and we made it through there in record time. One small scream, a "good sport" sticker, and off we went to Pratt 3 to see our new bedroom, which housed a total of five cribs. The other mothers greeted us and at a quick glance, I could see that their little ones were all in some sort of traction. I felt as if I was watching an episode of *MASH* but with much smaller bodies. As time went on, none of this fazed me.

Kevin came in for dinner and at that point I was relieved to see a familiar face. The nurses gave us a "show" on the Stryker frame, the apparatus that was to support Erin following surgery. This all made me a bit uneasy because I was finally beginning to process what changes postsurgery would bring to Erin's life, and I could feel a bit of a lump once again in my throat. Kevin seemed to do much better.

The Stryker frame was like no other piece of equipment I had ever seen. Essentially, Erin became the hamburger and the frame, quite literally, provided the roll. The staff would have to turn her over every so many hours and then take the top off and keep her strapped on the frame. This was a process that would continue after surgery and before casting so that her spine would have proper support. Needless to say, Erin was a bit small to be in a Stryker so it had its drawbacks and is not one of my favorite memories. Erin survived it all quite nicely but not without a few harrowing moments.

The night before surgery, I slept on a cot in the hospital conference room and was most appreciative of the fact that I had something flat to put my body on. I remember lying there thinking about the whole situation. I didn't really know why all this was happening. I felt very fortunate that I had had children at all. I also recalled that moment when Dr. Ramenofsky's facial expression had altered so quickly. In just one instant, your whole life can change. As parents, our natural inclination is to want to fix whatever is wrong, but that's not what life is all about. Life is good, but it is often not fair. That was one of the first lessons I had to learn. Once learned, it was never forgotten.

⌒⌒⌒

June 19 was surgery day and Erin and I were both up bright and early. At seven, they gave her the prep shot and ten minutes later she was on her way, ducks and all. Oh yes, those ducks, which looked like prime candidates for surgery themselves. The go-cart ride to the operating room was a little tense. Erin looked very suspicious; I think she was finally catching on. Saying good-bye was hard.

Shortly after 1:00, a nurse came out to report that they had removed the diastematomyelia (bone spur) and that Dr. Goldberg was proceeding with the fusing. I was relieved that the process was moving along as planned, but I really didn't know what this entailed despite what I had been told. It all seemed so complicated. I remembered that the fusing was as important as the removal of the bone spur, so I was pleased that they were now onto Plan B.

At 3:15 they called to say the fusing was completed. Because of what they found when they went inside, the surgeons had had to fuse five vertebrae instead of three. In addition, Erin had spiked a temperature and had some bleeding so they felt they needed to stop. All of this would ultimately extend her stay in the cast.

From surgery Erin went down to intensive care, where we were finally able to see her at 4:30. I had no idea what to expect and was shocked by all the apparatus. It would have been helpful to have some preparation for this world of monitors, tubes, and other medical paraphernalia.

This felt like the longest day of my life and looking back, I think it probably was. Erin had a very bad tape mark on her left cheek and ear but otherwise looked peaceful. A cool-mist mask covered her face and she was hooked up to a fetal heart monitor, all standard procedure. What really astonished me were the tubes that were draining the wound.

Kevin, who had arrived that afternoon, was more in control than I and able to talk to Erin. We stayed with her for nearly two hours. In those days, parents could not stay the night in intensive care. Since Erin was sound asleep, we decided to go home to the boys. I knew a change of scenery would be good and that Erin was in the best of hands.

The next morning Rose accompanied me to the hospital. I needed a strong soul by my side, but I didn't realize how hard it would be for her to see Erin in such a state. When we arrived, things were pretty quiet. Erin was beginning to feel the pain and discomfort that follows all surgery but is especially severe that first day. She had been moved from the bed onto the Stryker frame and looked like a peanut in a big shell. In spite of all her discomfort, she was doing well and because of this was going to be moved back to her own room. That meant that I could stay the nights with her; I was very pleased.

The ride back to Pratt 3 was very difficult for Erin as it would be for anyone less than twenty-four hours out of a major operation. You can well imagine how tender and sore that little back of hers was and I'm not sure how she was processing all this at such a young age. I was relieved when they finished settling her in and gave her a shot of morphine for the pain. Within a short time, all that discomfort subsided into a peaceful sleep.

I decided to take Rose home while Erin was sleeping so that I could be back at the hospital by the time Erin awoke. When I got back to the house, I was feeling very sad for the boys. In the days before the surgery, they had found a box turtle and in the frenzy of Erin's surgery, I had forgotten to bring it in from the little pool in the backyard the night before. Some animal had decided to have the turtle for its midnight snack and I was horrified to see what was left of the poor creature. I couldn't bear to tell the boys the truth because they were having enough trouble dealing with all the changes taking place around them. And I was angry at myself for not remembering it was out there. The boys were very sad when I confessed and I was feeling that I had really failed them. I was much harder on myself than I should have been.

After I got everyone settled and Rose was ready to get back into the swing of being the surrogate mom, I returned to the hospital. As I sat there in a chair thinking of our deceased turtle, Erin began to stir. Within minutes after she awoke, Kevin arrived. She was so happy to see him that she put her arms up for a hug. It really broke my heart because it was so hard to explain that we could not enjoy this small act of affection for a while. Kevin looked just as unglued. There really wasn't anything either of us could say that would make Erin understand, but we tried.

Erin remained sober during the days that followed. I would sit and read to her for hours. Most of the time she'd doze off and I continued to read to myself. Sometimes I could spark a giggle with her ducks, but it was always short-lived. At least once a day I'd lean over and have a heart-to-heart, attempting to explain why all this was happening; I believe she understood more than I realized. I used to tell her we were fixing a little problem with her back so she could run and play like the boys. I'd reassure her that it was okay not to be happy about all this, but that it would get better. The rebate to all this came years later. It is amazing how easily and how well Erin expresses her feelings today.

∞ ∞

Once Rose returned to New York my life changed drastically and I found myself on a sort of treadmill, going back and forth to the hospital, sometimes three times a day. Each morning I would get the boys off to school, charge into the hospital to see Erin, return home and pick up Colin at preschool, take him back into the hospital with me, return for Breen at 2:45, and back to the hospital with both boys to see Erin. Kevin would meet us at dinnertime, take the boys home, and I'd stay on, many times until 5:30 the next morning. I'm not sure how the boys or Erin ever survived this craziness but, apparently, they did. I was not alone in this madness.

The boys did pretty well in the hospital although Colin was often very quiet. Breen wandered around asking all the little ones if they needed anything and was able to rescue many dropped toys. When you're up to your elbows in orthopedic apparatus, it's pretty hard to jump down and pick up your matchbox cars or dollies.

In those days I never really gave much thought to Colin's silence but clearly I should have. I had so little time to reflect on anything. A few years later I realized that the whole hospital scene made him both nervous and nauseous. And there I was dragging him in everyday. Once I recognized the problem, however, I was able to talk to Colin and to reassure him that these feelings were both normal and understandable and that it was okay if he didn't come in to see his sister. Siblings often wonder if they're going to be next.

∽∞∾

About four days out of surgery (June 23, 1979) Erin was given a portable X ray, which showed her spine at a 28° angle, a big improvement from the 46° on the day of her procedure. We were thrilled with the improvement. Three or four days later she was to be casted. By that point, the intravenous lines were out and Erin showed excellent signs of grumpiness. Her appetite was back and anyone who can eat hospital food with that degree of enthusiasm has to be feeling better. A physical therapist came by and showed me how to perform the exercises that needed to be done on Erin's left foot in hopes of strengthening it and turning it out a bit. Erin really howled. All the poking and prodding was getting to her.

On Thursday, June 28, Erin was ready to be casted. I had no idea what this entailed, but I knew I didn't want to miss it. I arrived bright and early with camera in hand. To keep my own sanity and note Erin's progress, I was keeping a daily journal and taking pictures of each piece of the puzzle so that someday, when Erin grew up, she could piece it together and try to understand it all for herself. Often understanding fosters acceptance. I also felt that it was her life and she deserved to know everything about it.

The castings were real shows. The "cast" of characters who participated will always put a smile on my face and they remain some of my very favorite people. During the process Dr. Goldberg was quite relaxed and explained all that was being done. I appreciated how they tolerated my presence as well as my need to photograph the occasion.

Erin was excellent during all these procedures and there were many. For the casting, she was placed on a T-bar and then wrapped in plaster and trimmed; I would venture to say that it was a bit like being a living mummy. The cast on her torso extended all the way from her lower lip to her bottom. Since she was not toilet trained, we had to use several pieces of plastic to protect her cast. Keeping a diaper on Erin would be a challenge. They didn't come in extra, extra, extra large.

With the cast on, Erin could finally graduate to an apparatus known as a Bradford frame, a rectangular pipe frame with a sheet of heavy canvas stretched across. It was like she was being placed on the runway again, ready for takeoff. I couldn't help but think that in some ways we were going in reverse. Here we were, back on "angles" again, a place we had left only six months before when the reflux was resolved.

The next day Erin was given another set of X rays which showed that the curve had remained stable and looked good. But the Bradford frame was causing problems. Erin tended to slide and developed pressure marks on her fair skin. Without the frame, it meant that I'd have to improvise and find another way to keep her at the appropriate angle.

At this point I was beginning to feel the stress of having the boys at home and Erin in the hospital. The trips back and forth were getting to me and the juggling of schedules was like nothing I could ever explain. I felt like a vagabond and longed to be showered and in one place, if only for a day. Throughout all this the laundry was done at midnight and lunches at six in the morning.

Dr. Goldberg was a very perceptive man and figured out where I was at just by looking at me. He and Dr. Scott consulted and decided to let Erin go home early since everything seemed to be stable and she had been an excellent patient. It was time for me to handle the ups and downs at home. I felt so inadequate mothering the boys and looked forward to being at home with them full time again. Kevin's work schedule was overwhelming and even though he did hospital visits and got the boys off in the mornings, he really wanted everything to be the way it had been before. I also would have liked everything to be normal again, but I was slowly realizing that our definition of that term was going through a transition.

CHAPTER FIVE

Adjustments

∞

Erin's discomfort that first week home was greater than I had ever anticipated and clearly a learning experience for us both. The muscle spasms came frequently; I felt helpless. When they occurred, I would talk to her of silly things as a distraction; sometimes it worked. Those were the occasions when my crazy faces really came in handy. By dinnertime I felt like Jerry Lewis, except I think he had a lot more fun.

The visitors arrived nonstop and I was torn between needing a friendly face and a desire to hit the nearest pillow and sleep, sleep, sleep. The evenings were the hardest because by then I was thoroughly exhausted. For the first five weeks, Erin awakened several times a night. I used to sit in a rocking chair with her propped on two pillows so her legs would clear the sides, trying to hold whatever parts of her were free of plaster. The cuddling was tough but we managed.

One day I decided that Erin should be able to take walks just like other toddlers and I spent four hours rigging up the funniest contraption I've ever seen. Dr. Seuss would have loved it! It had sturdy baby-carriage wheels, a car-bed with an opening in the bottom for Erin's legs, and a stroller awning to protect her from the sun. Erin saw the last few minutes of progress and looked at me as if to say, "God, I hope she doesn't expect me to ride in that jalopy!" In spite of its shabby appearance, it was a means of transportation, and I regret that out of all my picture-taking during this time, I never took a photo of the "Erin-mobile."

When we went for walks in this contraption, people were speechless. If the mode of transportation didn't shock them, seeing Erin's sweet face in all that plaster did. For those who regained their composure enough to question her condition, I immediately responded, "Oh, just a little operation." I'd look down, give Erin a wink, and off we'd go.

By mid-July, the weight of the cast and the intensity of the heat revived Erin's reflux problem. Every meal seemed to come up as quickly as it went

41

down and cleaning it off the plaster and around her neck area was awful. Poor Erin must have felt so "gooky" and yet she was the only child I've ever met who smiled the entire time the vomit was pouring out of her.

I finally called Dr. Goldberg in hopes of a solution. He decided to make an opening in the cast for Erin's tummy to expand more under all the plaster. He also decided at this point to bivalve her leg cast so that I could begin the physical therapy on her left foot, weakened from circulation problems caused by the bone spur. The physical therapy would help lessen the disparity between Erin's two feet and eventually help her to walk with less difficulty. Needless to say, Erin was not at all thrilled with any of this, but we hoped the cast opening would resolve the vomiting problem and allow her to relax a bit more on a full tummy. Smaller but more frequent meals also helped.

Well, I knew it would take time for us to get all the bugs out and I can honestly say that there was never a dull moment. Every day was like a new chapter and the mystery of the unknown kept me in constant suspense. I was determined to try just about anything to keep both Erin and the boys smiling. Sometimes it worked and sometimes it didn't.

No sooner had we resolved the vomiting problem than Erin's ear infections returned. I brought her in to see the ear, nose, and throat specialist to drain her ear. He sent us on to a pediatric surgeon in hopes that we could obtain further insight into Erin's vomiting. The surgeon suggested even smaller portions at meal times and, when I left, I felt that I was going to be home feeding a bird.

That poor ear ended up needing to be drained one last time. Getting Erin into the hospital for these episodes was a real operation, if you'll excuse the pun. I had to fold down the back seat in the station wagon, prop her up in the car-bed in the back with a belt holding her in one place, and find a body to ride with me to serve as a cheering squad. At the time, I had a retired neighbor nicknamed Aunt Ruth by my children. She was always willing to come not only to my rescue, but to the aid of many other people as well. She'd hop in the car and entertain both Erin and me the whole way in. She has since passed away, but we have very loving and appreciative memories.

∞∞

Why, I'll never know, but in the midst of all these adjustments we decided to try our annual vacation week at Cape Cod. The boys needed a break and because Erin was being so good through all this, I think we really felt that we could pull it off. It was one of our poorest decisions. Never did I think about what 95° temperatures would do to this little plaster-clad body. We were unable to bring along the comforts of home: by the time you get a car packed for three kids and two adults, there is no room for fans, let alone air-conditioners.

The first few days went pretty well. Then, suddenly, the air temperature soared and Erin struggled. All of this set off her vomiting. I called the hospital to report the latest adventure and I think they were in disbelief that we had even attempted this excursion. They wanted to see Erin as soon as possible. It was obviously time to pack up and go home. It was difficult to tell the boys that their much-anticipated summer vacation had come to an end. But I wonder if they really even wanted this vacation as much as we thought. They were a bit confused but very cooperative. Their ability to adjust at times like these was amazing. They didn't express a lot of disappointment, but I am sure they felt it. They simply repacked what they had just unpacked and off we went. It was a much quieter ride home. Their frustration would surface later as almost a delayed reaction.

Once again, the pediatric surgeon was awaiting us, this time in the emergency room. He ordered a barium swallow to do an X ray of Erin's digestive tract. Erin had long since left the bottle so they gave it to her in a cup. Not only did she gulp it all down, she asked for more. How many kids request a second barium swallow? How we all laughed!

Erin was so good for the X ray that they rewarded her by taking a picture of her much-loved ducks. We still have the image; it's part of Erin's archives and the ducks now rest gracefully on the shelf of her closet enjoying a "bird's eye view" of Erin's life.

After radiology we shoved off to Pratt 3 once again. The room was becoming our "home away from home" and this time I was relieved to be there. Dr. Goldberg was already awaiting us. He felt that Erin's vomiting had been set off by a combination of things, but that she really needed to be back on the Bradford frame at an upright angle. He was right. In spite of all the little engineering features I had rigged up to keep her elevated, she kept sliding down in her bed. So, here we were, going in reverse again, back on the runway.

Since Erin was soon to need a new cast, Dr. Goldberg decided to get her stabilized and then proceed with the next casting, which was a piece of cake. Unfortunately, due to the intense heat and humidity, we had to stay on an extra day in the hospital so that the cast would be thoroughly dry. I would venture a guess that the materials they use today are much better able to adjust to these conditions. We were thrilled when the last section dried and we were once again heading home.

∞∞

The Bradford frame changed our existence considerably. It had to be placed in Erin's crib, which meant she had to spend many hours in her bedroom. At times, it was like being in isolation. I refused to stick a television in her room and was determined to stimulate her with books, magnetic letters and shapes, puppets, and anything else I could come up with. I didn't want her just to vegetate; I wanted her to feel that she was still part of the family activities.

For both Colin and Breen, the August of 1979 was a bust. It was a confining time and the house was often in a state of complete confusion. By the end of the first week I stopped making excuses and warned friends they had to enter at their own risk. Some did and wished they hadn't, some didn't and were probably better off.

As for me, surprisingly, I was comfortable with the chaos. I was able to accept the fact that beds wouldn't get made, dishes might not get washed, and that I couldn't satisfy everyone's needs the way I thought I could prior to Erin's diagnosis. Regardless of what others thought, I felt we were hanging in there very nicely.

The one advantage to the Bradford frame was that Erin was able to sleep very comfortably. She had been at that same angle as a baby and this time around it was much easier. In the afternoons, while she napped, I was able to devote time to the boys. Erin slept soundly from 7:30 at night until 6:00 the next morning, and I finally felt fully human again. I looked so much more rested that my own friends didn't even recognize me. One day, a dear friend babysat so that I could get out for a haircut. Upon my return, as I was getting out of my car, another friend drove past. Suddenly, she stopped her car, backed up, and yelled out the window, "Mary, is that you?" Obviously, for a time I had lost my identity. Thank God it was coming back.

Owing to the Bradford frame the vomiting almost completely subsided and Erin's ear infections also diminished. I was finally able to sit on the front step and, with the help of pillows, balance Erin on my lap so she could see that the world outside still existed. On one of those lovely summer days, while we were soaking up the sun's rays, a yellow jacket decided to crawl around my toes in my right sandal. Since I was allergic to the little varmints, you can well imagine how uneasy and relatively helpless I felt. Erin was pretty solid in her plaster and I was all of about 105 pounds. Even though my arms were as strong as any man's at that point, to get up with her from a sitting position took about five minutes and superhuman concentration.

For a long time I watched that damn bee in what seemed like a contest of wills. Suddenly it disappeared, and with a sigh of great relief I readjusted my very rigid toes and stiff foot. Then I felt the sting — the little devil had disappeared under my middle toe. I knew I was in trouble. Unfortunately, I was out of my antihistamine prescription and it was not being dispensed over the counter at the time. It had been fifteen years since I had last been stung, so I really was totally unprepared. I watched my leg double in size and by evening my shoe wouldn't get over my toes; not even a sandal would fit. The added weight of picking up Erin really made my leg ache.

The next day Erin was due for another cast change. As I look back, I'm not sure how I ever drove our car to the Floating. The pain from the bee sting had affected my whole body. I got Erin as far as admissions and then a volunteer ordered a go-cart from transport. She looked as if she wanted to order one for me, too. I will never forget how relieved I felt to arrive at Pratt 3 and know that the nurses could take over. They then called the emergency room and sent me down.

The doctor in the emergency room was terrific but quite firm about my letting the reaction go so long unattended. He sent me off with some meds and said it would be a good five to seven days before the swelling went down and that I was to try and stay off my feet whenever possible. Easier said than done.

By the time I returned to Erin, the nurses were waiting to tell me that one of her ears looked infected again. They had already bivalved the cast and she was resting on the shell. It was clear that the specialist was needed. The nurses gave him a call and before long he arrived and had everything under control.

The idea of Erin's getting yet another new cast put me in a very upbeat mood because it meant we were one step closer to the end. You tend to play these games, counting on every event you can that will help you feel that progress is being made. Erin's back had remained stable and we seemed to have the other problems under control. Even though her left foot lacked an ankle reflex, we had that in hand, too. I continued the physical therapy on her foot daily. We were finally halfway there.

Simultaneous to Erin's admittance, I had taken Breen to Massachusetts Eye and Ear Infirmary for a tonsillectomy. Poor Colin must have really felt left out; either that or very healthy. When Kevin arrived home that evening, he went over to Mass. Eye and Ear and stayed the night with Breen, and I eventually went home to Colin to relieve the babysitter. I clearly remember that day because Kevin and Breen watched Carl Yastrzemski get his 3,000th hit for the Boston Red Sox. The things that stand out in our minds!

The next morning, Erin stayed on at the Floating while I discharged Breen from Mass. Eye and Ear. Kevin had gone to work and Colin was tucked away in school. Breen and I then returned to the Floating for Erin's discharge and once again, our medical wagon headed for home.

∞∞

The rest of September went by very quickly. The boys were into school full swing and I had finally settled into a routine with Erin. Her days seemed to go by with relatively few complications and I even got in an early morning shower. For sure, we lived a fairly isolated existence. I longed for the day when Erin could get out and roll around like other children her age. For her part, she found innumerable ways to entertain herself. She had every reason to be cranky and difficult, but I don't think that this was ever part of her character. That remains true today.

Dr. Goldberg was extremely pleased with Erin's progress and allowed her to sit, propped up with pillows, in a bounce chair. With all that plaster, there really wasn't a lot of bouncing going on but it was great to see her holding her body erect in a kind of sit-slouch. Finally, she could see her food again. We were all pretty excited.

I made a special effort each morning to get to the front step so that we could wave good-bye to the boys as they boarded the schoolbus. I'm sure the kids were told some pretty bizarre reasons for why the boys' sister was so covered with plaster. Whatever version they recounted, the bottom line was that they could talk about it. That was so important to me because I wasn't able to participate in their school activities. At least the other children could see that we existed.

Having little time to tend to my own needs, I ended up with a bad cold but eventually rallied and got Erin to the Floating for a cast change as well as the long overdue removal of her papilloma. I distinctly remember how excited she was when I put her in the car onto her frame for the trip; her cabin fever must have been worse than mine. Before we knew it we were back in our old room. The first thing Erin did was look around and check out the "inmates." I found myself looking to see which one had a mom in tow, a comrade, someone with whom to share a cup of coffee.

On that particular day, with a cold in full bloom, I was really looking for relief. I still felt lousy and I just wanted to go home and find a bed. I was also a bit worried about being in a pediatric unit and spreading my germs. Since there were no moms around, I shared my concerns with the nurses and they were probably very relieved when I left.

At home I lost track of the time and twenty minutes after I arrived the doorbell rang and the boys were standing outside with big smiles. The kind of "Oh boy, we have mommy to ourselves" smiles so I knew I was not long for the couch. We went off to get an ice cream and a bit of togetherness, the best medicine of all for me.

∞·∞

When I returned to the Floating, a Dr. Peace was in the process of bivalving Erin's body cast. I'm not sure which was scarier for her, the noise or the thickness of the dust. To top it off, as the nurse began rubbing down Erin's skin in preparation for the new cast, she discovered a heart-shaped button that had been missing from Erin's bathrobe. As you can imagine, it had created a very gooey, messy-looking sore. I felt terrible. I thought I had removed everything, but obviously I didn't do it soon enough. The things that no one tells you when you have a child in a body jacket. Remember to remove all buttons on clothing. Immediately! Today, I could write the book. Well, actually, that's why I'm writing this book. Erin still sports a tiny indentation on her back which, if you view closely, looks just like a tiny heart.

My night's sleep seemed like a cat nap. Since Kevin was away on business, a former babysitter came over early and stayed with the boys so I could get in to Erin before she had anesthesia. When I arrived in the morning, Erin had already had her sedatives, but was awake enough to see me.

Shortly after, Dr. Goldberg appeared and together we discussed that Erin's left calf and foot were still not up to snuff. There was a definite difference in her shoe sizes not to mention that one leg was chubbier than the other. It was at this time that Dr. Goldberg mentioned the possibility of Erin's walking with a limp. I had learned there are tradeoffs, and I was so excited at the thought of her finally walking at all that the possibility of a limp was not of immediate concern. Overall, Dr. Goldberg felt that things were moving along on schedule.

Erin's surgical procedure went fine. Dr. Ramenofsky removed the papilloma and implied that this growth and the previous one had perhaps come from Erin's biting her cheek when she went to sleep. As I processed his remark, I remembered that her mouth did move when she dozed off. She definitely had my genes — never an inactive moment, not even in sleep.

The doctor doing Erin's plaster sculpturing with Dr. Goldberg the next morning certainly enjoyed Erin's cooperative spirit as well as his own craftsmanship. After he molded the cast to her little body he drew buttons and a skirt, then proceeded with the leg cast. It was so funny to watch and still serves as a good example of how they tried to make Erin's experience an upbeat one. It could have been rushed, intense, and very impersonal, but instead it was pretty amusing, most especially for Erin. As we left, Dr. Goldberg indicated that we were probably going to need only one more heavy cast and then a lightweight version as a transitional mold. Time had become our friend again.

Going home was especially exciting because Kevin had spent the week wallpapering our extra bedroom so that Erin would now have a proper little girl's room. With what little spare time I could find, I had put the finishing touches in place and found the whole project a nice diversion.

It was clear to me that my two wonderful boys were absolutely off the wall and not so wonderful, their typical behavior when I returned from a hospital visit. They certainly let it all hang out. Finding the energy to deal with them at these times was like looking for a needle in a haystack. Even today, when I speak to other parents who have a child in the hospital and others at home, I find that this circumstance continues to serve as a point of frustration. Finding the energy to please everyone is not easy. Nobody seems to have found the answer, but the stories that are shared are pretty wild.

To top it all off, we were four days away from Halloween. The boys had decided to carry a bag around for Erin — God knows what their explanations would be to all the people who answered their doors to two anxious boys and three trick-or-treat bags. They had their own way of representing Erin's situation; some days it was their sister who looked like R2-D2 (from the *Star Wars* films), other times it was "our sister who's all wrapped up like a mummy," and finally, there were the times when they forgot all about her. As I look back I can recall how important it was for us to find humor in our predicament and the boys always seemed able to do so. They still do, though at ages twenty-two and twenty-five, their sensibilities have advanced to a whole new level.

CHAPTER SIX
Ups and Downs

∞

As November began, I could finally see Erin's frustration at her immobility beginning to surface. Her back was healed and she was feeling well. As a result, she was much less willing to nap. She had slept enough in those first months after surgery to last a lifetime, and she was ready to be fully involved again; that's pretty tough with plaster all over your tummy.

At this time Erin had a dear friend named Lara who was a favorite source of entertainment. Lara would stand on a chair next to Erin's bed and keep her giggling. It allowed Erin a view of the world from a perspective she could relate to, which was very, very important. That wonderful friendship that began at the side of a crib continues today.

Although Erin couldn't break any records physically, her vocabulary and ability to speak, in full and well-put-together sentences, was exceptional. She had an almost exaggerated intonation if she was in her room alone. I'm sure she was cleverly using that tone to get one of us to drop in and visit. You know what? It worked. Yet Erin was also very tolerant of being alone. If you indulge your child to extremes when they are in these situations, the future may present you with a very demanding result. You can be sensitive and caring without spoiling them.

To help occupy Erin's time, a business acquaintance of Kevin's had sent Erin storybook tapes and a tape recorder. What a great gift. For part of her waking time I would play a story. Sometimes I would make tapes with my own special brand of animation, and I think Erin rather enjoyed hearing her mother, "the nut," on tape. When all else failed, out came the non-toxic markers and she would go to town on her cast while I held the mirror so she could witness her own artistry. I would never recommend allowing a toddler to do this unattended. But I must say that those markers were often the highlight of her day. Underneath all our smiles, and most especially

Erin's, was a family that longed to see her rid of all this and leading a "normal" life.

I could no longer prop Erin up on pillows and know that when I turned my back she would be in the same position. Despite the weight of the plaster, she had mastered turning over on her tummy and her expressions of surprise and victory were wonderful. Of course, once over, she reminded me of a turtle that didn't have the energy to get on with it. Seeing her getting stronger and more mobile warmed my heart and made the days pass by more quickly.

But each time we went two steps forward, we always seemed to go one step back. Just before Thanksgiving Erin started another deep chest cough. I called Dr. Abelman and he came right over to check her out. Did I say check her out? It was pretty tough hearing a chest through a tummy full of plaster. Just in case we were onto something big, he put her on medication, rolled his eyes, and said "Keep smiling!"

∽∽

On December 3, 1979, while the rest of the world was going from store to store trying to finish their last-minute Christmas shopping, I was admitting Erin for what I truly hoped would be her final cast change. Dr. Goldberg had indicated during the previous casting that perhaps we would need only one more. Although I always felt bad about Erin's going back into the hospital, in some ways, it represented progress and so I tried to make it one more adventure in our "How to Get Yourself 'Back' Together" saga.

For the fourth visit in a row, Erin was placed in Pratt 301. As always, there was a new resident, part of the routine in a teaching hospital. The big changing of the guard occurs on July 1, so I always made sure that if Erin had a procedure, it wasn't around this time, although I'm sure it might have worked out very nicely. As the others before him, the new resident had the honor of unveiling Erin's small body from the big, clumsy plaster shell. On this occasion it was obvious that it wasn't Erin that was nervous, but the doctor. This resident talked to her the entire time he worked. To help him out I kept her as distracted as I could. Finally, it was time for the unveiling and as with all the others, there was a surprise awaiting us: tucked down inside the cast, creating a very nasty sore, was Erin's missing yellow Snoopy pencil. I had searched her room for it for days. Little did I know that she had it all the time. Once again, we will never forget this remnant of her childhood since it left Erin with a lovely little scar to add to her collection. The only person who looked more shocked than I was the resident.

My greatest thrill at those unveilings was being able to hold Erin using the shell of her cast to support her back. As with many good things, just when we were beginning to feel cuddly, it was time to twist her around in X ray and see how things were going "back" there. I wouldn't know the results until the next morning, but it was then we would find out how successful the fusing had been.

⌒⌒⌒

When I arrived the next morning Erin was a bit of a grouch, which was very unusual. She was starving and had not been allowed to eat before the casting, so she wasn't a particularly happy camper. Brigitte, the assisting nurse, finally got a few smiles out of her and more or less took over for me while I anxiously awaited Dr. Goldberg. I depended on his reports for information, as well as some much-needed support.

He finally arrived absolutely beaming. With delight he announced that Erin's spine was solid and holding at 26–27°. I had a great urge to grab Dr. Goldberg and give him a big hug, but I figured the technicians might get the wrong idea, not to mention Dr. Goldberg's reaction. Perish the thought that they see my nutty side. Today, a bit more carefree, I'd probably show them that aspect first!

Discharging Erin that day made me quite emotional. I was naive enough to think that it might be Erin's last overnight in the hospital. And a small part of me thought that we might be rid of her scoliosis at some point in time. I had so much to learn and to accept, but like most things in life, there are steps to go up and I kept thinking that we were much closer to the top than we really were.

For the first time in months, Erin left the hospital in a carseat, looking a bit like a stiff, but still far more normal than during the previous departures. We even had a prescription for orthopedic shoes and the promise that Erin could join the ranks of other toddlers and sit in a stroller each day. I was really on a high until I looked into my rearview mirror and noticed that Erin had either poured a gallon of milk over her head or vomited most of her lunch. Obviously, she did not share my enthusiasm for the carseat. Rather than go back into the Floating with Erin dripping and looking like a reflux ad and chancing the loss of our new carseat privileges, I cleaned her up as best I could. I made it home in record time. I had learned to "go with the flow" and on that particular day, that is precisely what I did.

When we got home I cleaned Erin up a little better and off we went to Belmont's Family Shoe Store. She and I were a pretty rowdy pair when we

51

got excited and I'm not sure that the saleslady was prepared for us that day. The poor woman could not figure out why any mother could be so happy with a baby all wrapped in plaster. Then she saw that Erin's left foot wasn't the same as her right and that really made her curious. She didn't just look, she studied us, hardly able to take her eyes off Erin. I tried to allay her concerns and gave her a brief insight into our situation, but then she got even more upset so we basically bought the shoes and hustled out the door.

From there we proceeded to the Filene's department store for a proper snowsuit for Erin to sport during her walks in the stroller. Up until this point we had been outfitting her in oversized hand-me-downs from a dear friend, a great savings for us in both time and money. This was the first attempt at beginning a wardrobe for Erin and I was very excited. Thank goodness the lady in Filene's didn't really get a chance to scrutinize us very well. We were out in a flash.

We had lots of good news to tell the boys when they got home from school that day. As always, they wanted to know when Erin was going to walk, the question on all of our minds, and I was feeling quite optimistic.

∞ ∞

As a result of the lighter carapace, one of the most exciting changes in Erin's life, as well as mine, was our return to daily walks. For both of us it would become the symbol of mental health during our day. If you can remember back to the beginning, we really didn't have a stroller anymore because I had turned it into something that only Rube Goldberg would appreciate. Now it was time for us to get a new model that was a little less embarrassing to be seen in. I needed to find one that was wide, light, and compact, one that would finally give my back a breather: it was really starting to ache from carrying Erin so much.

I decided to "schlepp" out to the Toys R Us store in a neighboring town, as I had heard that their selection was the best. I was also looking forward to Erin's reaction at seeing a real toy store. As always, there was one complication that I had not anticipated: Erin would not fit in the seat of the store carriages and she was far too heavy to carry. She had already surmised the situation and looked at me as if to say, "Now, what do we do?" While I explained to Erin that I thought we had a minor problem, the whole aisle of people turned around and stared. Finally, a salesgirl solicited the store manager, who was very accommodating. He brought over five strollers and before long we found a good fit. There are advantages to looking so needy.

The next few days Erin and I were almost religious about our walks and the boys loved being back at the park on a regular basis. We got a lot of stares but by this time, I was prepared and I think Erin was, too. Unlike a broken arm or a broken leg, what Erin was modeling, although hidden under a snowsuit, was a bit overwhelming for some. I understood that and at times it was necessary for us to move along quickly. I'm sure I offended a few moms, who continued to fire questions as we hurried along, but I had to protect Erin. The very last thing she needed was a replay of her medical history. She had to live it, but she didn't have to hear it.

Lara, Erin's good buddy, was wonderful and it was nice for us to arrive at a door that didn't ask a lot of questions. I would often share my frustrations with Nancy, Lara's mom and a dear friend, and explain that a simple walk just wasn't that simple. It was the little changes that were often the most puzzling to me. I was beginning to understand what I had been told by parents of special-needs children: they would often remind me that we were part of a world that placed far too much importance on perfection. Finally, I understood what they were saying.

☙❧

The combination of the cut-back cast as well as the success of the fusions allowed Erin the opportunity of becoming more mobile. During the weeks that preceded the holidays, she adapted herself to crawling all over again, working very hard at pulling herself up on her knees. Her arms were very strong and it was amazing that she could haul herself up with a tummy full of plaster. I had to be careful not to let her overtax herself, so I made sure there was a balance between her active and inactive periods. At times, she wasn't too thrilled about sitting still and I couldn't blame her one bit. But I didn't want her to strain herself and Dr. Goldberg had said to monitor things so that they did not get out of hand.

Although I was still physically and emotionally exhausted, the pressure seemed to be lifting as Erin's options were finally increasing and her life was "moving" along quite nicely. And I was, once again, able to satisfy the needs of the boys, which made a big difference in my daily routine. On the surface the two appeared patient and yet I suspected that they were somewhat frustrated because of my lack of mobility. When Kevin traveled, it was very hard for them because there was no relief. It was hard for me as well. They used each other to vent their frustrations and some of their fights were worth the price of admission. I would watch them totally overwhelmed, wondering if I had failed as a mother. In reality, with or without Erin's condition, they still would have had those skirmishes.

Erin loved the constant activity of her brothers' friends coming in and out each day. They would often stop to marvel at her body sculpture and add their own prognoses. We had a lot of future doctors in those days and some very funny stories about their own so-called "sick" family members. I loved all their tales, and Erin was thrilled with the attention.

The fact that it was December and Erin was creeping along over rugs once again made it seem as if for an entire year, time had stood still. It had been exactly one year since Erin had been able to come off the "runway." At that point her gastroesophageal reflux had subsided and we really felt that we were coming to the end of her health problems. Unfortunately, it was the end of one but the beginning of another. That's one of the things I've come to learn about congenital scoliosis; it's really the sum of many parts. One thing seemed to lead to another and some of her really serious concerns were often masked by smaller, more minor maladies.

In the midst of all the other goings-on in our house, Christmas of 1979 was right around the corner. I had always loved the holidays but this particular year, I found the time a bit oppressive. Feeling exhausted, I wondered where I was going to get the energy to pull off being Santa Claus. I was also in a real dilemma trying to think of gifts for Erin, who kept asking for riding toys. I wasn't sure how to respond. She certainly wasn't ready and I wasn't sure when or if she'd be up on her feet. We had already bought out the bookstores.

For the boys, who were bouncing off the walls in anticipation, the shopping was easier. On Christmas morning it was as if their eyeballs had springs as I watched them scoping out one another's gifts while trying to open their own. Poor Kevin looked pretty depressed as he perused the corner of the room that had the toys that needed assembling. Normally, Santa Claus does it all ahead of time, but this year we had a different agenda. The following Christmas we made sure we bought only preassembled items.

For Erin, all the excitement and activity was a bit much, and I wasn't able to devote as much time to her eating schedule as I normally did. As a result, she spent a good part of the day vomiting her meals while harboring yet another cold.

Well, we survived the holiday chaos and life settled down considerably by December 27 to be quickly replaced by another event that in my mind was much more exciting: Erin had stood up perfectly erect in her bounce chair without support. She looked just fantastic. The boys and I cheered so loud that you could have heard us in Boston's Back Bay. She was able to balance herself in that position for at least a minute, which she had never done so well prior to her surgery. We called Kevin at the office and, I'm sure, brightened his day.

This event marked the beginning of a really great vacation week. I got a babysitter to stay with Erin one day and I was finally able to spend some time with the boys. I was concerned about how they were doing and needed to let them know how much I wanted to be with them.

New Year's came and went and we managed to do some entertaining. At that point, I had "cast life" down to a science. As for Erin, she had mastered toilet training, letting me know when she had to go. Once her cast was cut down, I was able to hold her on the toilet. I was amazed she didn't crack the seat; when the cast met with the porcelain it made quite a bang and Erin would let out a big giggle. It would have made a great cartoon. I was truly amazed at this latest accomplishment. It involved as much time, if not more, than the diapers, but it was so important for Erin to feel that control over her own body.

CHAPTER SEVEN

A New Year, A New Life

⌘

We had apparently survived 1979, some of us in better shape than others, and were now just a small step into 1980. I prayed that I would never again see a year like the past one. I can only imagine what Erin might have said.

My first lesson of the new year had to do with Erin's cast. As a routine I used to stick my finger in between the cast and Erin's body. If it didn't fit, the cast was getting too tight. In light of this, on January 4 I decided to call Dr. Goldberg. When they had done her previous casting, they had also made a mold for a lightweight model and I was anxious to hear if it was ready. The thought of something that was removable was very appealing.

On January 9, 1980, Erin finally escaped from her plaster for good. She still hadn't walked.

It had been almost ten months since all of this madness had begun, although to me, it seemed more like ten years. I had learned more about the people around me than I had or would at any other time in my life. The bond between Erin and me was a solid one. The boys had been wonderful brothers to her and more and more I realized that they were the most normalizing element in her life and would remain so as Erin developed into a young lady. We were very lucky to have them.

∞∞

The adventures were not over yet. Our next would be in South Boston with the orthotist who would be making Erin's lightweight jacket. He would also have the pleasure of uncasting her. Did I say pleasure? We'll see.

The shop was remarkable. There were artificial body parts everywhere and the background music was the sound of the machinery that created them all. I admired the craftsmanship and skill that allowed people with disabilities the assistance they needed to engineer their way through life. It was an amazing place. Totally distracted by what was before me, I had forgotten how concerned I was about getting Erin's current cast off. There was not one centimeter of extra space between the cast and her body and I had anticipated some difficulty getting her out. I knew that both Erin and the orthotist would have to be very steady. The noise of the drill would be the worst part for her, and for him, it would be having a very steady hand. If he could pull this off, it would be a major miracle.

Well, don't you know, there are no miracles. We did fine from under Erin's arm to her chest but then, without warning, Erin suddenly moved and the drill grazed her skin, leaving behind a nice, clean, half-inch slice. She had been so perfectly still until this point that both the orthotist and I stood there motionless, dazed by her sudden movement. The orthotist was devastated and reassured me that in twenty years, this had never happened. It was clear to me by his reaction that he was sincere in his words. What amazed us both was that Erin never cried. It had happened in a split second and neither of us panicked or made a big deal of it. We simply controlled the bleeding with tissues as best we could, and quickly finished the job of uncasting her. Once again, we found another missing object in her side, this time a yellow crayon. Unfortunately, it left an ugly and gooey sore which the orthotist said we could address when he finished.

After the fitting we called Dr. Goldberg to share our horror stories and arrange for him to see Erin immediately. We said our good-byes to the orthotist, who still looked very upset about the cut, and then found our way to the Floating. Erin was in a great mood and not the least bit unnerved. Dr. Goldberg was delighted to see the lightweight jacket and I almost felt like we were making a social visit. His very calm, confident, and sincere manner was comforting and reassuring. He examined Erin's new sores and supplied us with a list of instructions. He suggested butterfly sutures for the drill cut, explaining that they would pull it together nicely. He gently cleaned out the gooey little crayon sore and announced that we would have yet another indentation to remind us of these days. As I drove home, Erin dozed and I finally was able to enjoy my own quiet celebration of this new phase.

That night we celebrated with pizza, including Erin in our feast. After dinner, while she was being royally entertained by her brothers, I removed the Bradford frame from her crib. After I put everyone to bed, I went back and looked in on Erin and continued to do so for at least three hours. She was sound asleep.

Erin navigated well with the lightweight jacket and was far more mobile than she had been a year before, prior to her surgery. She crawled with great ease and speed and was able to stand up beautifully, holding on to a chair or table using her hands for support. I could always hear her when she got down because there would be a bit of a thump as her body made contact with the floor. In the quiet of a moment I would think to myself that if we hadn't had a calendar to remind us that this stage had taken twice as long to arrive at, it would seem as if the past year had been merely a dream.

On one particular afternoon in mid-January, when Erin was supposed to be napping, I heard a very loud and extremely happy little voice. It did not seem to be coming from a child who was lying down. I tiptoed up the stairs and there was Erin standing up in her crib, very proud of her accomplishment. I called to the boys, who gave her the audience on which a toddler thrives. It was Breen who soon realized that she couldn't seem to get herself back down. The bounce in the mattress was like standing on a waterbed for Erin. Breen stood there with her for a good hour, patiently assisting in her new venture.

By the next day, Erin had mastered the whole process and was ready to conquer yet another frontier. I could clearly see that at any age, the human body really does naturally progress from stage to stage. Piaget was right when he said that each stage builds on and is a derivative of the accomplishments of the previous one. Normally, children progress through these stages so quickly that we don't allow ourselves the time to process the events. Why would we need to?

♋

On Monday, January 21, 1980, Erin and I once again set off for the Floating. I always looked forward to these visits, as I said before, because they served as my barometer. Drs. Goldberg and Scott were the only ones who really knew where we were going with all this or I should say, where they hoped we were going.

"Hello, young lady," were always Dr. Goldberg's first words to Erin as he entered the examining room. He would sit down right next to her and say, "Well, I'm very glad to see you" and she would beam. Despite her age, both Dr. Goldberg and Dr. Scott kept Erin involved in this process. It was as if I was just a fly on the wall. This made me feel so good.

At this appointment Dr. Goldberg was especially pleased to see Erin standing. After a thorough examination, he sent us off, two very happy people, with his sanction for Erin to have a bath, the first one since June of

1979! When I think of all the crumbs that used to sneak down her cast as well as some of those other surprises, I can almost feel the discomfort myself.

This visit with Dr. Goldberg was significant for other reasons as well because he had given Erin his blessing to move ahead. Things seemed to be back to "almost" normal. I would still observe her cautiously, but certainly with more comfort than before. I guess Erin was a better listener than I thought because that very evening she crawled up the living-room stairs to the second floor. By the time she reached the top she must have been exhausted because she lay flat on her tummy and put her head down. What a creative way to get a child tired enough to nap, I thought to myself at first. But I soon realized it was simply a brief respite. The trip down was a bit threatening and so she gave out a hoot for some fast assistance. It was very funny to watch. The boys became a captive audience and brought her down so many times that they finally ran out of steam. Eventually, Erin conceded.

∽∾

By the time Erin's second birthday arrived on January 31 she was moving around like a bulldozer. Nothing seemed to stand in her way and because of her adventurous spirit, she was covered with bumps and bruises. I never left her alone in a room because there was no warning to her falls. She was a master at crawling to a table and whacking her head as she attempted to stand up. In the beginning, I followed her around, hovering over her, until I finally figured out that this was not normal and that Erin would be just fine. I was the insecure one.

By Erin's second birthday, I could hold out my hand and if she had something to brace herself with on the other side, she could eventually let go of the support and accompany me around the room. The crucial part was maintaining her balance. She seemed to have her own way of reaching her goals and I truly believe that at that young age, she really did have goals. The gross motor progress came steadily and was not compromised by any new problem. That was certainly a first for us.

Erin's second birthday party was small since our house seemed to be in the throes of a major flu epidemic. There was not a lot of singing, nor did Erin's birthday cake go fast, but she didn't seem to mind one bit. We certainly made up for the lack of festivities in later years.

Not long after, I found myself writing in her journal less and less. I had started writing that very first day she was diagnosed, March 22, 1979. The recounting of events had served as a form of therapy. Perhaps I'm just a visual learner or maybe it was a way for me to go back and process something that I found so hard to believe. I know one thing: my reaction was normal and not unlike that of many others. I needed to find some means by which to put it all in perspective and that vehicle turned out to be my journal. I realized that if I didn't write it down, the years would fly by and I would never remember with the same detail. As Erin became more active, time became an increasing challenge and I often had only a minute to jot down a few notes. But what I didn't get down on paper, I would store away in my mind until some later date. Eventually, it all got recorded.

As things improved for Erin, I became more and more anxious to read about congenital scoliosis. Again, the paucity of material was very frustrating. I knew that some of what I had learned with Erin were insights that could apply to any family whose child had problems that required tending. The cast experience alone was an eye-opener: so many little details that one would never have thought of beforehand unless you had someone or something to teach you.

To help us, Dr. Goldberg had recommended *Deenie* by Judy Blume, a story about a teenager with scoliosis. Although the book was a far cry from our predicament, it did give me some insights into what adolescence would be like for Erin. There was also a wonderful book by a woman named Rosalie Griesle entitled *The Crooked Shall Be Made Straight*. Rosalie, now an adult, had had many fusions even as an adult, but has been able to live a full and normal life, not without incident. Hers was the story of struggles amidst much happiness. To me, its strongest messages were acceptance and perseverance. I regret that this book is now out of print. It really helped me to understand that scoliosis doesn't go away; it's with you for the duration. Rosalie's writing really opened my eyes to what our "tomorrows" might be.

ᔉᔊ

February seemed to fly by. Erin continued to make her way through our house with great determination, but did not seem to be making progress toward walking alone. If her balance was not absolutely perfect, she would sit down and revert to crawling. She seemed to know her limitations and there was no way of enticing her. It's amazing how much like that she is today. It's so out of character for her to be impulsive; spontaneous, yes, but not impulsive.

Erin's godmother, Rose, had again come for a visit. It was wonderful to have an extra set of hands "and then some" since Rose had brought a friend along. Her visit was especially uplifting for me since she hadn't seen Erin since June and could really note the progress. It was a great time for us all and allowed me some time to be with the boys.

Just when I was feeling confident about where we were, Erin plowed her way down six hall steps. I was numb. I knew I needed to calm her down so that I could see if there was any damage. She just seemed to lose control and I was too late to break the fall. The solidness of the body jacket made it hard for me to grab her and I was afraid if I grabbed her arm, I might break it. I called the hospital immediately. Off we went. She was checked thoroughly and sent home.

On March 5 it was back to the hospital again for a checkup. Dr. Goldberg was pleased to see her moving around so well, but surprised she wouldn't let go and walk freely with a hand for support. She just didn't seem to be able to maintain her balance. I was concerned, but he was reassuring and said that if she still did not let go in a few months, there were some tests that could be done. He sent us on our way saying, "Let's just let nature takes its course and see what happens," some very sound advice.

⁓

A few days later we decided to bring Erin and the boys up into a part of Belmont known as the "open space." Erin had never seen anything so wooded before. Altogether the area consisted of about a hundred acres of ponds, woods, walking paths, and plants, affording us the opportunity to simply drive a few miles into nature's backyard.

For me it was like going home to the country atmosphere of Connecticut where I had been raised. I spent most of my youth in Redding, a beautiful town that had been protected from developers by strict zoning laws. It was where Mark Twain had lived as well as many other interesting people who wanted to escape from the hustle and bustle of city life. I had spent much of my time there tramping through the woods, catching bullfrogs, and bringing polliwogs home in a jar.

Accompanying us on this outdoor adventure was Breen's dear friend Jason. The two boys thrived in the woods and recycled anything they could get their hands on to create squirrel traps, snake sanctuaries, and everything else that appealed to their imaginations. Erin was so distracted by the environment, which was so rich with diversions, that she let go of Kevin's hand and managed to cover a considerable distance holding on only to me. At first the accomplishment didn't even register until I realized that Kevin was several steps ahead of us. It was nice for Kevin to see one of her milestones firsthand. If only we could program our little ones to perform after the parent gets home or do "instant replays." Today, the wonders of the video world have surely capitalized on this. Soon Erin was really cruising along. She had mastered getting off the potty chair alone with no remarkable injuries and, even though she still needed a hand to hold, she moved along with great ease.

For a while I had been leaving Erin with a wonderful woman named Helen Austin two mornings a week to get some space for myself and provide Erin a much-needed change of scenery. Helen, who had no children of her own, had been both supportive and loving to Erin and was much more than a babysitter. She was one of Erin's favorite people in the world. Helen's apartment was small, simply furnished, and wonderfully homey. She had a collection of unique toys, which her husband had made years earlier. I could understand why children loved to play there. Helen was aware of Erin's status and her difficulty in letting go and walking unassisted. Helen was a private person who often processed your concerns and then spent her own time working on them constructively, either in her mind or in any other way that was appropriate and helpful.

At the time, I was leaving Erin with Helen to go to a lecture series on Thursday mornings at McLean Hospital. I would drop Erin off at about 9:15 in the morning and return around noon. On that particular day, almost one year after Erin's diagnosis, Helen answered the door glowing, but without Erin at her side. I questioned her and she abruptly replied, "Well, just a minute now, I'll have to find her." "What a mood change," I thought to myself; so unlike Helen. I stood in the living room patiently waiting for almost five minutes. Finally, Helen returned and asked me to give Erin a call. I thought she was really losing it. "Hurry up, Erin," I beckoned, "we have to go home and eat lunch." Suddenly, this wobbly little body approached me ever so slowly and with such calculated steps that it looked as if she was moving in slow motion. I was both thrilled and amazed at how steady she appeared. Helen, much like a fairy godmother, was quite pleased at what her magic wand had accomplished.

∞∞

Having Erin walking really changed the dynamics of a day. She moved around like a little robot and when she became tired, she literally plopped down wherever she was, waiting to be recharged. It took me about a week to understand that when she dropped, it was only a temporary state. Once Erin was fairly steady on her feet, we widened our horizons and spent at least two hours a day at the park. There, Erin thrived on the climbing toys and, at the age of thirty-plus, I found myself going up slides, sometimes in the wrong direction, to ensure her safety for the trip down. Although my friends were impressed with my equanimity, inside I was in turmoil as I processed some of Erin's activities. I learned I really had to "grin and bear it" and simply allow Erin to be Erin.

Her only enemy was the impulsiveness of other toddlers and their friendly shoves. Not at all a physical child, Erin was very poorly equipped to respond. She still hadn't mastered the balance necessary for these unannounced pushes. I saw a few of the mothers do some fast talking as they sized up the situation. Eventually Erin figured it out and a good, hard stare seemed to get the moms of the shovers to redirect their little ones to another victim. Erin was clearly able to fight her own battles.

At this point things were moving along pretty normally and for the first time in over a year we would be bringing all the troops together for Breen's First Communion. Unfortunately, church never seemed to have much significance in Breen's life, and I was hoping he wouldn't decide to share any of his seven-year-old insights with the priests. Religion to Breen was being a good boy and playing with his trucks. I'm not sure he was any different from a number of other children his age.

We really had a houseful that weekend and I had them sleeping anywhere I could possibly fit a sleeping bag or a pull-out sofa. It was fun to be celebrating, but a lot had changed in our lives. I made sure that the focus remained with Breen. I wanted him to have a wonderful, wonderful day. And he did.

During the weeks that preceded Breen's celebration, Erin progressed beautifully. She had integrated herself nicely into the park and met lots of new friends. The boys enjoyed the opportunity to resume normal schedules again and for the most part we lived like any other young family. The boys were good to Erin and she enjoyed watching them do all the crazy things two active little boys do.

On May 12 Erin and I returned to Dr. Goldberg. She was two years four months old, and it had been eleven months since her fusions. She was wearing her "total contact" or lightweight jacket full time. For the first time in quite a while, Erin cried at the sight of a doctor. She was obviously feeling normal and not wanting any more prodding or poking. But they were a necessary evil. I could tell that Dr. Goldberg was pleased with her walking although he did note her clumsiness, which I had noted as well. He seemed fine with it all and decided to wean Erin away from the lightweight jacket four hours a day and then, eventually, six. This was great news. I could also start her in a swimming program. And last but not least, we had graduated from orthopedic shoes to the real McCoys. All this in one visit.

CHAPTER EIGHT
Return to Normal

∞

By the summer of 1980 Erin's life was almost normal and as important, so was life for the boys. The stress of the hospital stays was behind us and we seemed to be like any other family. I signed Erin up for a special swimming program at a YMCA and plugged the boys into summer camp.

Erin loved the swimming program and we made the acquaintance of another mother and daughter from our town. The program opened the door not only to swimming and a new friendship, but above all, to a new independence for Erin.

That year we spent ten wonderful days at Cape Cod. Erin's removable jacket was not a problem and we learned how to adjust her beach play to jacket-free breaks. I was religious about keeping track of her time and keeping her jacket clean and away from all the sand. After the Cape, we went off to Connecticut to visit my grandparents. They were a great welcoming committee. My grandparents were both thrilled and amazed at Erin's progress. I'm not sure at eighty-plus years they fully understood what her birth defects entailed, but I knew one thing: they made the kids and us feel terrific. They were able to block out all the negatives and simply enjoyed life, and most especially each other. I had a hard time processing their ages and the fact that they might not have that many years left. Little did I know that my grandmother would live to the ripe old age of ninety-six and my grandfather nearly as long.

∞∞

Near the end of the summer Erin and I were off to the Floating once again, with a more cooperative Erin this time. Dr. Goldberg measured her back and watched her walk, looking pleased with her progress. I gave him a brief update of what life was like at home and was thrilled to hear him explain to Erin that she could graduate from wearing the jacket during the day to a reduced schedule at night.

The new regime worked out well and I watched Erin master many things during those last few weeks of summer: her mini-wheels, going up and down the big slide, climbing around our jungle gym (with lots of supervision); the list went on and on.

On September 24, Erin went for her second casting for another jacket to fit her expanding little body. She was a bit nervous at the onset, but Dr. Goldberg allayed her fears and it was over in a snap. Within a week, the orthotist had her new jacket ready and we were off. Our schedule was a busy one, a result of many of her medical issues. I found it hard to imagine being a working mother and pulling off this program, although I knew many, who did. I stood in amazement at their ability to get it all done.

∞∞

It had been almost eleven years since Kevin and I had had a vacation alone other than a night here and there. He had a stress-filled career to contend with and you already know how I had been spending my time. When the opportunity came for Kevin to attend a conference in San Francisco that fall and to bring me along, we decided to go for it. Some very dear friends, Dee and Erich Ippen, offered to take the troops — all three. Their youngest son, Jason, and Breen were the best of friends, as they are today. Colin was flexible, and Erin, although in need of watching, was also pretty easy. In spite of my optimism, as we ascended the airplane I felt Dee and Erich deserved to be canonized. It was the nicest thing anyone could have done for us. California was wonderful, but being away was the best. I can't stress enough how important it is to get away, alone, even if it's just overnight. Although it's never easy organizing for these events and you do worry, it is such an important break for both you and your little ones. They need to know they can survive very nicely without Mom and/or Dad.

As for the Ippens back in Belmont, I'm sure they were counting the days until our return. Caring for your own two children, plus three more, one of whom has a medical record, is truly an example of two very selfless people. We hoped we would return in time to save the friendship.

By the sixth day, we were both getting anxious to get home and see the kids. They have a way of growing on you and it's hard to break the habit. As the airplane landed in Boston, Kevin and I took one look at each other as if to say, "Here we go again!" We knew we would not have a moment's peace again for quite some time. And we weren't too far off target. The minute our car pulled into the Ippens' driveway, out came the troops "loaded for bear." Dee looked like an exhausted version of the Pied Piper. She helped us get the kids' belongings into the car in record time and, I'm sure, reconsidered ever making such an offer again. On the way home and on into the night, we got a detailed description of the entire week. At times, if the stories were accurate, I was amazed that Dee and Erich didn't turn to drugs. It certainly cured me of ever considering more than three kids.

After that, we went non-stop into Halloween and then into the latest in flu epidemics. I don't think the two were related, but regurgitated candy leaves much to be desired. I eventually hid all the goodies and became the least popular mother on the block.

Erin's flu hit her body like a ton of bricks and seemed to settle in her bones. For one entire day she made no attempt to get up or walk and I must admit, I overreacted. Those were the times that I really appreciated Dr. Goldberg's prompt attention. He explained that it was simply the route this particular strain of the flu was taking and suggested I wait a few days and see how she fared. He was absolutely right and the change in Erin was extraordinary. Had she not had her birth defects, I don't think I ever would have gotten so worked up. I had to learn that since she had orthopedic issues, achy flus might perhaps have a more pronounced effect and it might take a bit longer for nature to take its course. None of us moves around very quickly with a bad flu. There was always a new lesson to learn.

CHAPTER NINE
Transitions

∞

Toward the end of November, when Erin was once again back on
her feet, I set out to find a preschool for her for the following fall.
I had researched several programs, but they were concerned about
the liability of having a child with Erin's disability. I really didn't think of it
as a disability and felt uneasy with their reactions. I needed to be able to
trust whoever was going to be in charge of Erin and above all, I needed to
feel that she would be safe.

A good friend had suggested the Eliot-Pearson School, which took in a
variety of children and had been one of the first lab schools in the U.S.
After its founding as the Ruggles Street Nursery School and Training
Center in Boston in 1922, it was now located on the campus of Tufts
University in Medford. If it was anything like the Floating Hospital, which
was also a Tufts affiliate, I knew I would be happy with the care.

I spent a wonderful morning at Eliot-Pearson and made an appointment
to return with Kevin. I was impressed not only with the staff but with the
philosophy of the school as well, which was very supportive of
mainstreaming. It warmed my heart to see physically challenged and
developmentally delayed children in the same classes as the so-called
"normal" kids. I felt confident that this would be an excellent placement
for Erin and regretted that the boys had not had an opportunity to
experience such an environment.

The holidays came and went very quickly. Kevin's mother came up from
New York and braved colder temperatures than we had seen on Christmas
Day in years. She was to be commended for making the trip in such cold
weather and for surviving the week without earplugs.

January of 1981 brought a job transition for Kevin: after several years of
handling real estate investment for a large Boston insurance company, he
decided to move on to a smaller firm that allowed him more opportunity

for growth. For me, the most important piece to all this was that we could remain in Boston. Leaving the supportive medical environment of the Floating Hospital would not have been easy and, a part of me felt, very unwise. Erin's medical situation was unusual and there were no guarantees we would find another team that would be as invested in her as Drs. Goldberg and Scott. The change would have come at a very difficult time.

January flew by and before we knew it we had a visit from Erin's godfather, a priest from Michigan, a lot of fresh snow for everyone to enjoy, and a fair amount of ice-skating for the boys. Suddenly, it was January 31, 1981, and Erin was enjoying her third birthday with her own little circle of friends. Life was going full-speed ahead.

⋘⋙

After Erin's spine surgery we had promised the boys that as soon as she walked, we'd book a trip to Disneyworld as a treat for their being such supportive brothers. Had she not walked within a reasonable period of time following her surgery, we still would have taken them; I made that clear from the very beginning. So, with Erin mobile, we were able to make good on our commitment.

On Friday, February 13, truly a lucky day for our clan, we boarded the plane for Orlando, Florida, where we met my parents, who had taken adjoining hotel rooms in an effort to help us out. If the boys wanted to go back into the park with us at night, my parents were there to get Erin into bed.

From Disneyworld we went on to Busch Gardens, where Breen convinced me to accompany him in a boat that went along a water route, somewhat like a roller coaster. I was not in a normal state of mind when I agreed to go and I was almost catatonic when I got off. I haven't been on a ride with him since, nor do I intend to ever again. From Busch Gardens we visited Sea World and it was at that point that I remembered that Kevin was leaving me with these three very excited children to go on a business trip that overlapped with our family vacation. My parents and I were dividing up the troops and driving to Miami to have a visit with my grandparents before our departure for Boston.

The ride from Orlando to Miami with three kids coming off the most stimulating five days they had ever spent was indescribable. It was the last time my parents ever made such an offer. We had a record visit in Miami and before I knew it I was standing in the Ft. Lauderdale airport with three very tired children awaiting a flight that was overbooked by thirty people. When the ground attendant offered me four tickets to anywhere in the U.S. if I'd take the next flight, I looked her straight in the eye and said, "Do you have these fantasies on a regular basis?" She laughed and boarded us five minutes later. Little did I know we would have a two-hour wait in the airplane, on the ground, without benefit of air-conditioning or meals.

∞∞

By late February, Erin was in need of a few minor alterations to her bivalved jacket. Her appetite had increased so much over those last few months that she looked about to burst her seams. And so, on March 12, we were off to the hospital for yet another casting.

Before we knew it April had begun and the weather was giving us a sneak preview of spring. For about a month I had been contemplating moving Erin into a bed since she was getting so active in her crib, torn between providing her with more independence and comfort and the sadness I felt knowing that I was putting the crib away for the last time. I had thoroughly enjoyed our babies and saying good-bye to those days was like closing a chapter in my life, one that I had only just begun. For Erin, who had been constricted by her medical issues, going from the crib to the bed would be much like getting out of jail. No more being strapped to a mattress at an angle, no more Bradford frame, no more plaster casts; finally, a new lease on life in a better location. Erin loved her new bed and I would sneak in several times a night to check out the tiny little body that appeared lost on this big, flat surface. And there, tucked under each arm, were the ducks.

Easter was upon us and we no sooner finished our holiday festivities than we were about to embark on yet another move. This time, a bit bigger than the transition from crib to bed. In late winter, shortly before Erin began to walk, we had purchased another home in Belmont. It had taken us some time to find one in the same school district since we didn't want to make the boys change schools. They were happy where they were and we wanted to minimize the disruption of moving as much as possible.

The house itself was a clone of our old one but much larger and in a location that, in later years, would be more convenient for the children, as they could walk to the three schools they would eventually be attending. I had the task of getting much of the work done. The diversion was both delightful and distressing. Satisfying the needs of several different sets of workmen, each of whom had different tasks and deadlines, was not always easy. In between contracting, I still had to get the boys to summer camp and take care of Erin, so I didn't have a lot of time to dwell on the issues of getting the house in shape.

I remember going to an office party with Kevin at the time and being asked by a woman who worked with him if I was "just" at home with the kids or if I worked. She made being at home seem like a trip to the spa and I was so aghast that I merely replied, "Right, I'm just at home with the kids!"

Whatever you want to call it, life was pretty busy and the emotions of the boys were all over the place. Leaving our old street was much harder for them than I anticipated. For me, saying good-bye to all our special friends and neighbors was equally hard, since I could no longer walk across the street and find them within arm's reach. They had been a wonderful support system for the children and me and many scenes flashed through my mind as I prepared for the move. My friend Nancy, who had moved with her family to a larger home shortly before us, used to come down and help me turn the encased Erin upside down to wash her hair. We would laugh hysterically not only at the process but at the expression on Erin's face. My other friend, Merry, was like a surrogate mom to our boys and always returned them to me with a smile and a story. To say that the boys felt right at home at her house was an understatement. Then there were all the other neighbors, each of whom had played some role in the children's lives.

Moving day was July 10. The boys thought the van was awesome and experienced the thrill of waking up in one house and, some fourteen hours later, going to bed in another. I felt that I was once again ending one chapter and beginning another. Kevin looked as if he had one continuous Excedrin headache and I'm sure he wished he were back in the office. A new house is nice, but, at that moment, it was hard to get too excited.

The first several weeks at our new home were rather hectic. Never before had I been surrounded by so many men at such an early hour. The work was an ongoing saga and there were lots and lots of surprises, such as the day we attached the washer hoses only to find that five minutes later my laundry room was flooded from pipes that went nowhere. Erin's schedule was totally off, and I found it a challenge simply getting her fed and dressed. The one dividend to the move was our new little next-door neighbor named Danny. Although a year older than Erin, he was the perfect playmate and kept Erin content and active. She had given up on me.

The boys, who went off to camp each day, were thrilled with their new home and the location. They had the third floor all to themselves and were really in their element. Over the years, they were often too much into their element such as those times we spied water balloons and fireworks sailing out the third-floor windows. For the lady across the street, observing our show was better than watching her TV. The action was live and the boys were always available for autographs afterward.

Just when I thought the transition to our new home was behind us, Erin became difficult and wanted no part of her brace, something I had not anticipated. She was beginning to notice that neither the boys nor her friend Danny had to wear one and began waking two or three times a night. She would sit up in bed, tugging on her shirt to get her brace off complaining, "Take this thing off!" Her other famous line was, "It's too tight!" It was not an easy time and continued for about six weeks. Perhaps it was her way of reacting to the move. I think she was overwhelmed by all the changes and I didn't blame her one bit. The bottom line was the brace had to stay on.

⌒⌒

As Erin began to improve, the thought of her ever having another operation hung over me like a cloud. I had almost convinced myself that we were just about out of danger. Dr. Scott had seen her on July 28 and was pleased with her progress. That look of concern he once wore was nowhere in sight. He had her stand on her toes, at least to try, and tested her reflexes. He didn't remark on anything in particular, so I felt confident that Erin was right where he had hoped she'd be. He even took a picture of her feet. Erin appeared flattered and, I must say, it was a first for me. Dr. Scott also showed me the slides of Erin's surgery, which I greatly appreciated. I wanted to know everything I could get my hands on about what was wrong with Erin's spine. And although I was able to grow and understand more because of people like Dr. Scott and Dr. Goldberg, even they couldn't answer many of my day-to-day questions because they hadn't lived with it themselves.

Before I knew it, the summer was winding down and it was late August. Erin's soon-to-be preschool teachers from Eliot-Pearson stopped by for a home visit, which impressed me and delighted Erin. This would make her transition easier for she was now at least a little bit familiar with her teachers and, likewise, they with her.

The boys started school the Wednesday after Labor Day, which was the traditional time for most public schools in our area. While Erin waited in anticipation of her first day at preschool, she managed to master tying her shoes. Her fine motor skills had always been exceptional and these tiny little fingers manipulated the laces like a pro in slow motion. She would sit for long periods of time trying to tie them, so I decided to give her a few lessons, never dreaming that she'd stick with it. Those shoe laces entertained her for the greater part of that day. Such perseverance.

On Friday, September 18, 1981, Erin began nursery school. She was thrilled to go and I was amazed at her comfort level. As luck would have it, Erin's wonderful transition to nursery school was short-lived and as the weeks passed we had many a tearful morning. She had spent her first few years in a relatively protected environment and was perhaps a bit intimidated by the activity level of her classmates. Both of these issues were normal; Erin would eventually adjust if I didn't get gushy and allow her to "wimp out." The children who were active were merely being normal preschoolers. Erin was in excellent hands, which I was able to observe for myself. To buffer my own issues of letting go, I picked up a small tutoring job in my school system, which served as an excellent distraction. It was nice to have some breathing space, and it was really wonderful to be around adults again.

On October 5, Erin and I set off for a visit with Dr. Goldberg, who noted no remarkable changes in her status. Erin's X ray was excellent and her spine was holding at 26° with full mobility. She still dragged her left foot a bit but Dr. Goldberg maintained that we should wait and see. I remember that visit so well because after Dr. Goldberg gave Erin her glowing report, he said, "Well young lady, what is it that you'd really like to do?" Erin's response was, "Play hockey," which sent Dr. Goldberg and me into instant laughter. Older brother Breen played hockey at that time, so why not the same for Erin?

☞☜

The fall of 1981 seemed to fly by and I became known as "taxi Mom," a title that I had managed to shed during Erin's convalescence; it was now back to reality. Soon we were in the midst of the holiday season once again, complemented this year by some wonderful snow.

Erin continued to progress and our March 1, 1982, visit with Dr. Goldberg was glowing. He still wanted her to wear the jacket as a precaution and so a few weeks later we went back and had another mold fabricated. In late spring Colin made his First Communion, helping to maintain our good status within the Catholic Church. In addition, I continued to run a Saturday special-needs program for the diocese so that these children could receive their sacraments.

While the boys were still tucked away in school for a few more weeks, I spent some time researching something that was at the very top of Erin's wish list, ballet lessons. Now I'm sure you're wondering the same thing that I was at the time: how the devil is this kid going to pull off all those positions with her fusing and a weak left foot? Had I been just a bit more insightful, I should have realized that this issue was mine, not hers. If she wanted to do something, somehow she'd figure out a way to do it. After some research, I contacted a well-respected ballet teacher, explained Erin's situation, and arranged for her to do a few private lessons as a test run.

Fortunately, Erin's good friend Lara agreed to do the lessons too, so it was a nice little summer adventure for them both.

In addition to the ballet, Erin had become a real water bug and by the end of the summer she had pretty much mastered the dog paddle. The boys, who were excellent swimmers, became her teachers and their sometimes overzealous presentation was a good reason for Erin to learn how to swim sooner rather than later.

She had also started in a preschool piano class begun by the mother of one of her classmates from Eliot-Pearson. Laurie, a concert pianist and vocalist herself, gave the children an excellent introduction not only to the piano, but to the world of voice and music as well. It also provided Erin with another opportunity to be with her peers. For certain, she was having a wonderful summer and a life rich with good experiences.

CHAPTER TEN

Crossroads

∽

At this point I was approaching that dangerous crossroads that many of us come to after a successful outcome and a return to a normal life. At times, I really believed that Erin's back problems were going to go away and that we were really home free, with the exception of her wearing a brace as a precaution. It had been more than eighteen months since Erin had come out of her plaster cast and the world was being very kind to us. I felt very, very lucky.

Then one day I noticed Erin limping a bit more than usual. I figured it was my own insecurities and that really everything was just fine. As the weeks passed, what had begun as merely a glance had expanded to my actually studying her use of her left leg on a daily basis. Was I becoming neurotic? Was I finally going off the deep end? I really wondered.

Finally, in late August, it was time for a visit to Dr. Goldberg for a checkup. I shared my concerns and he suggested recasting Erin's left foot since the heel cord or Achilles tendon was still very tight. The new removable leg brace was exactly like the one she had been in during her convalescence from surgery. From my perspective it was a bit of a setback, since it meant we were adding to the apparatus again.

We left the office with a daily physical therapy schedule. In addition, Dr. Goldberg pointed out that we would have to buy two pairs of shoes each time we went shopping since the brace would increase the size of Erin's foot. I suppose I could have minimized the effort and gone back to orthopedic shoes but, had I been in Erin's position, I would want the kind of shoes the other kids had. And so we ended up with a "dinghy" on her left foot and a "canoe" on her right.

What was hard to accept was that the door which I had almost closed behind me was slowly opening again and the message, though subtle, was that it wasn't over yet. Such a difficult reality for a parent to process when really all you want for your child is a chance for them to follow their dreams, hopefully without baggage. But the door began to open wider and wider and Erin's limping advanced to tripping and falling and, at times, completely losing her balance. What was so difficult was that others did not notice. Finally, in late September, I went to her nursery school teachers for input. At first, I think they really wondered about me since Erin had started off so well. But by the end of the third week, they, too, could see the difference. My emotions went from concern to relief and then back again to concern.

On September 21 I decided to call Dr. Scott; I sounded so desperate that he saw me the next day. I just couldn't imagine what had happened to bring about this weakness. It was clear that Erin also knew something was up and she was very quiet and subdued when I announced our visit. Dr. Scott was delighted to see Erin and very gentle as he examined her. He noted some progressive turning in of her left leg and a more pronounced inversion of her left foot than during previous visits. After he poked around for a few minutes, we returned to his office to go over her status. He said that he would review her records in the event that he had missed a tethering band or a thickened filum or connective tissue (both of which can cause spinal problems) and then give me a call.

Most of this was Greek to me but, at the time, my mind was so preoccupied and clouded by my concerns that I probably was only capable of processing about 50 percent of what he said anyway. I was beginning to see the big picture, and it was very different from the one I had filmed in my mind. It was time to leave the fairy tale and move on.

For the next two weeks, we watched Erin very carefully. Then Kevin caught me in a weak moment and I agreed to drive him to New York for a business convention, visit his mom and Rose, and then drive home alone with the kids. Remember, after Florida I had said "never again." But we had learned to grab whatever time we could with Kevin and so off we went.

It seemed that we were down and back in a flash. A nice breather from our usual schedules. I no sooner walked into our house than the phone began to ring. It was Dr. Abelman, our pediatrician, announcing that Dr. Scott wanted to do another myelogram on Erin. Apparently, after reviewing her records, he noticed that she had a thickened filum and that she also might have had some tethering as a result of scar tissue from the previous operation. The filum, which acts like a shade pull, is located at the bottom of the spine and apparently was causing some tension in the spinal cord, which affected its function. When I finally reached Dr. Scott on the phone, I had only one question, "Would it mean more surgery?"

Getting Erin in for her myelogram was easier said than done. She had picked up a serious cold that had settled in her chest and getting her well enough to go under anesthesia took almost six weeks. Finally, on November 9, 1982, we checked in. Finding an empty bed was a real challenge. Eventually, we got one and found ourselves in the accommodations of the new Floating Hospital, which had just opened its doors.

For our boys, this was a particularly difficult time. I would once again be the "absentee landlord" racing between home and hospital. Kevin was so immersed in his job that we had become ships passing in the night. At times he looked absolutely exhausted and there just never seemed to be time for him to rest. Our dear friend Rose in New York sensed my need for another pair of hands and agreed to come up and help us out. What would I have done without her?

Erin's hospital roommate was a lovely Spanish girl about thirteen years old. I spoke almost no Spanish and she no English, so you can just imagine the gesturing and facial expressions. Even Erin got into the act; it was pretty funny to watch. In the midst of our attempts to communicate, the third-year medical student assigned to us entered the room. Both Erin and I took a double-take as we both realized that she was bound to a wheelchair. "What a fabulous role model," was my first thought as I watched her handle Erin. It wasn't easy reaching over the bed and completing a successful exam, but she had it down to a science; it was quite impressive to watch. She talked as she worked and explained to Erin why she was in the wheelchair and even shared with us that she was from a neighboring town to Belmont. I still see her from time to time and always get a good feeling when I think back to that day. It really put some things in perspective.

The anesthesia team arrived next and expressed concern over Erin's cold. No sooner did they go out the door than neurosurgery arrived to draw blood. I was amazed at how Erin could cry without moving a muscle — such control. She even managed a smile for the technician as he left, probably more than I would have been able to muster up at that point. And just when we thought we were finished with visitors, Kevin arrived — but he came without apparatus.

That night I slept on a cot in a room adjacent to pediatrics and, by seven o'clock the next morning, Erin had had her sedative and was on her way for a CT scan and a myelogram. By dinnertime we were back in her room and I could hear Dr. Scott talking to the nurses. I was less receptive than I thought I would be when he announced that Erin needed more surgery.

Out of the corner of my eye I caught the expression on Erin's face. Dr. Scott tried to explain what was happening. Apparently, Erin's spinal cord was split more than they initially had anticipated. Just as he had suspected, at the bottom was a tethered area and, in addition, a thickened filum. The procedure was not as serious as the first surgery and Dr. Scott felt that Erin would do fine and be fully recovered in four to six weeks. Maybe!

Just as Dr. Scott was leaving, Kevin returned to the room and I was delighted that he could hear it firsthand. He had been much more optimistic than I that surgery would not be necessary, so it was best that he talk to Dr. Scott in person. Kevin accepted the results of the tests and, like me, was relieved that it would not involve a plaster cast. This time around it was all neurosurgery.

Erin was really losing her cookies following the myelogram and I was beginning to wonder if they had planted a little motor in her tummy that was dredging out all the extras. The intravenous line was a permanent acquisition and we weren't making lots of progress.

In the midst of all this Dr. Goldberg arrived and added his commentary on her status, sharing with me that both her back brace and leg brace should probably stay on indefinitely until we saw how things worked out. In his usual casual way, he waltzed out the door smiling, reassuring me that it would all work out. I spent that night in a wooden chair next to Erin's bed.

Promptly at 7:15 the next morning Erin and I began our trip down to the operating room. Erin was not a happy camper, but she had her own way of dealing. There were never any tears, just a hug, a kiss, "I love you," and my traditional, "See you later, kiddo." The quicker the exit, the better for everyone. Kevin arrived to warm the bench with me.

At eleven o'clock Dr. Scott came out to say that all had gone well. Just as he had expected the filum was the problem as well as some tethered nerves. He also noted that there was spina bifida in the lower area of Erin's spine. By definition, spina bifida means split or open spine, but Erin's was "occult," the mild form that can be seen in perfectly normal children. Also, instead of using stitches they had stapled Erin's incision closed as it made for a neater scar. The cosmetics of any surgery often play a more significant role in your life as you mature and become aware of every imperfection in your body. Although the thought of stapling skin really blew me away, if the final product was a better look, then it was worth it. Erin had a long life ahead of her.

By 1:30 P.M. Erin was down from the recovery room and, although somewhat groggy, was doing just fine. As she became more conscious and able to focus, the anesthesia began to wear off and her pain became more apparent. As soon as they gave her a shot she was not only more comfortable but able to use her bedpan. But there was a difference this time around. Erin was older and could verbalize her discomfort and seemed to be unclear as to why she was back in the hospital having another operation and why as she put it, "It hurts a lot." As a parent, you feel like a real creep when you're so healthy and your little one is feeling all the pain. And for Erin, the pain the second day was worse than the first. Kevin and I did shifts so that at least one of us could drop in on the boys. Erin was in no shape to see her brothers and, at this point in time, it would have been unwise to let them see her either.

By Monday, November 15, the crisis was over, so I thought, and Erin was improving. She ate well and looked much better. Dr. Scott even felt we could go home within the next few days. We had instructions for bed rest since that is how a surgery like this heals. Trying to keep a four-and-a-half-year-old in a bed all day would be a real hair-raising experience, but Erin was pretty easy to reason with. We also had a new physical therapy program for her left leg. Once again, our plate was full.

⋘·⋙

Within a few days Erin was home. Rose, who had come up to tend to the boys, was back in New York, and I was once again the charge nurse. As always, there was the usual entourage of visitors, but this time I really had to limit the time. Keeping Erin in the bed was quite a feat; I never read so many books to a child in my whole life. I had several of them memorized by her second or third day home. In desperation, I would dress up and act out some of the stories. Whatever seemed to work, I did.

On and off, Erin complained of headaches and when they came, they were severe. I called Dr. Scott and we explored a number of avenues of relief, some of which worked; the pain continued nonetheless. Dr. Scott and I talked daily and sometimes when he called, the noise level in the background was so high that I'm sure he wondered what was going on. Erin's friends were regular visitors and even though the volume was high when they arrived, the visits were brief and just what Erin needed.

Finally, we were scheduled to go in to get her staples removed. My list of concerns had increased on a daily basis: she had headaches, appeared more tilted than ever in an upright position, and her gait looked worse. All of these things might be absolutely normal after a surgery such as hers. I simply needed to be reassured. But the more I thought about the whole picture, the more uncomfortable I felt. I decided to ask Dr. Scott to give her the once-over before we went off to get the staples out.

A wonderfully perceptive and sensitive person, Dr. Scott was most accommodating and at a quick glance, agreed that something didn't look right. He brought Erin into his examining room and ever so gently removed the dressing that was protecting her incision. What a disaster. The incision had filled up with spinal fluid and looked very, very sore. Dr. Scott shared our concern and explained that our spinal cord is covered by a thin, balloon-like material called the dura. Somewhere in Erin's dura there was a pinhole leak that was allowing the fluid to escape. No wonder Erin was walking all bent over. Her discomfort was most apparent.

Unfortunately, Dr. Scott needed to drain that fluid out of the incision. As the parent, I wanted to give him my back instead of Erin's. Aware of my concerns, Dr. Scott called a few residents in to help hold her and asked us to leave the room. The sound effects answered my curiosity as to whether or not the procedure had been started. I was beside myself but there was nothing I could do.

⬥⬥⬥

Erin's stay continued right up to Thanksgiving Day. The draining subsided and I found a wonderfully supportive physician's assistant who kept me abreast of Erin's progress when Dr. Scott wasn't around. Since we were once again in the midst of another holiday, the hospital floor was pretty empty, so the nurses spent lots of time dropping in and keeping Erin comfortable. Thanksgiving arrived and we were given our walking papers but not without one last procedure, the removal of the staples. It certainly made for a tearful departure.

Our Thanksgiving that year was quite memorable. I have never stuffed a turkey and gotten it into an oven so fast in my entire life. The scene in my kitchen was like one of those old-fashioned silent movies. Lots of action — no words. And by seven o'clock "most" of us sat down to enjoy the first Thanksgiving we had spent by ourselves in years. As for Erin, she ate her turkey dinner "à la stomach," lying on a mattress which we had brought down and placed on the dining-room floor so that we could all be together. We all giggled at how funny our Thanksgiving scene looked, but in truth, we had much to be thankful for.

The next day Kevin's mother arrived on the scene to give me some help. I desperately needed some assistance keeping Erin flat as well as fulfilling the needs of the boys. She had not seen Erin and the boys in quite a while so she was anxious to come visit. Well, I must say, Granny came through "big time" and I think she left my house with a real appreciation for how complicated life becomes when you have small children and one of them is not well. She became my biggest fan and even mastered getting Erin on and off a bedpan. I became very close to her during this visit and saw a side that she had never shared before. Unfortunately, she passed away less than a year later.

During the weeks that preceded Christmas, Erin progressed nicely. The only evidence of any difficulty were some recurring nightmares in which she dreamed that they had not gotten all the staples out. I ended up buying a big mirror and showing her that area of her back to allay her fears. Eventually, she believed me.

In early December it was time for a visit with Drs. Scott and Goldberg. The latter observed the indication of a new angle to Erin's back; this time it was leaning to the left. He took three different angles of X rays to be sure, but there was no mistake, we were dealing with more curving. Sometimes I felt as if each time we made progress on one front, we starting losing the battle on the other. It was clear that she would have to get back into her body jacket the moment she was healed.

⌗⌗·⌗⌗

The beginning of 1983 was a wild time in the Mahony house. Kevin was working nonstop and the boys were hanging from the rafters. It felt as if their energy cells multiplied on a daily basis while I think mine had gone to sleep. And Erin, good as she was, had also changed. She had lost her innocence and become not only streetwise but somewhat of a worrier. I could certainly relate to that and, for the first time in months, I stopped writing in my journal. The revisiting was simply getting too hard.

Soon the school year was over and another summer was before us. The boys attended day camp for the month of July while Erin just "vegged" out with some friends. She was finally back to her old self and it was nice to see her relax and enjoy herself. And there was a lot to enjoy. That summer began with a new puppy and ended with a wonderful trip to California. Erin was once again thriving and it was clear to me that Kevin was hopeful that the worst was over and it would be clear sailing ahead. I envied his level of confidence but in my heart of hearts, I knew better.

Our vacation had barely ended and it was time to get everyone ready for "back to school." Erin was particularly excited since she was about to begin kindergarten. Colin was entering the fourth grade and Breen was beginning the sixth grade in middle school.

On the first day of class, Erin marched into Ms. Butler's room very confident that she was going to have a wonderful time. The school principal had been apprised of Erin's situation and made sure she wasn't being placed in a class with any kids who had severe acting-out problems.

Otherwise, there were no modifications to her day. School had been a wonderful time in my life and I think I was probably as excited as the kids on that first day. Erin never even looked back to say good-bye; she was far too excited.

The time did not go quite so smoothly for me and, I must admit, it took me a while to believe that kindergarten would be easy sailing and that we were out of the woods medically, at least for a while. Finally able to breathe, I took a job as a tutor, which seemed to fit nicely within everyone's schedule.

As we got more and more into fall, I noticed Erin's limp had once again increased and met again with Drs. Goldberg and Scott. Apparently, her second operation had affected the left leg, which is the chance you take each time you go in and do more surgery in an area like the spine. Our only recourse was to have her go back into her leg brace during the day.

Erin was not at all happy with having visible baggage again, and I completely understood. Several kids asked questions and it was hard for her to answer them since I don't think she completely understood it herself. I gave Erin an honest response when she asked me about it. "Yes, people will notice, but they would probably notice the limping more without it. In time, we hope, it will be easier than it is now and unfortunately, you really need it."

The positive side of the brace was that it helped Erin a great deal and her gait showed much improvement. She needed her teacher's help getting her left shoe on and off, but everyone lent a hand and it worked out just fine.

The holidays came and went and we had finally crossed over into 1984. Off we went north to the slopes to try to improve our very marginal skiing abilities. Erin found it difficult not joining in, but it was the one sport that the boys dearly loved and we had to meet their wants and needs, too. Fortunately, as Erin grew stronger so, too, did her options, including skiing.

Soon it was spring and then summer, with everyone involved in a variety of activities, including a family trip to Canada — the longest car ride in history.

CHAPTER ELEVEN
An All -Too -Visible Means of Support

⌦

Before I knew it everyone was back in school and life was on schedule. Colin was beginning his last year of elementary school. Because of their age difference, he and Erin would never be in the same school again. He was an excellent brother and walked her back and forth faithfully every day. Erin was now a first-grader and seemed to be adjusting well to her teacher, Ms. Brady. The support we received from Erin's elementary school was most extraordinary. Kevin and I will always be indebted to each of her teachers, as well as to the support staff, for all their help.

I took a job as an aide in the special-education department at Erin and Colin's school and decided to pursue my certification in special education, which had been interrupted after Erin's diagnosis. I worked half time, which still allowed me to continue volunteer work. Kevin was traveling 40 percent of the year so the job helped me retain my sanity and it gave me something to look forward to each day. Most important, it kept my mind off Erin.

In late fall it was once again time for Erin's checkup. Everything seemed to be stable and holding. The fusion was solid, and she would continue to wear the jacket at night and the leg brace during the day. Dr. Goldberg even said we could allow her to learn how to ski with moderation and a lot of supervision. She had mastered the riding of her two-wheeler over the summer and her level of determination at anything athletic was something to witness.

I called around to several ski areas searching for a good ski instructor who was familiar with physically challenged children and would be sensitive to Erin's situation. Cindy Gardener up at Attitash in New Hampshire came highly recommended. So, off we went for Christmas vacation week. If Erin had never shown an interest in learning how to ski, I can honestly say that I never would have pursued it. And in pursuing it, I harbored some pretty heavy concerns. Cindy was the one who really made it all happen.

Erin's first day was a disaster and quite rough on her body. Cindy took her off the slopes early and shared her concerns with me. My inclination was to bag the whole thing, but Erin would have no part of it. I thought long and hard and realized that Erin had a long life ahead of her with scoliosis and if I kept pulling her out of activities, it would be a long and uneventful one. Cindy never anticipated this kind of a response from me and I'm not sure I did either. She agreed to hang in there.

The next day Erin taught us all what determination is really all about. Within the first three hours she advanced from the beginner to the intermediate slopes. Cindy had a terrible time convincing her to come in for lunch. Erin had her own unique style, which looked a bit uneven from behind, but Cindy had taught her how to adjust her balance to her tilt and it worked just fine. The one drawback was the chairlift: if it came in too fast Erin would not have time to get on, let alone get safely off. We simply made a deal to do a lot of gesturing to the chair operator and hoped that he or she would get the clue. They did, and today Erin is an excellent skier with the form and confidence that many physically normal skiers lack. I certainly can't keep up with her.

∞∞

Erin's second-grade year started off so easily that it seemed like a continuation of the previous one but with a new teacher. The leg brace no longer posed a problem and her classmates were used to seeing her wear it. I continued to be "taxi mom" and spent much of my time transporting the three to soccer, swimming, and tennis lessons, and if I even anticipated a free moment, someone filled it up before it ever became a reality. Since my own mother had worked a good part of my life, I had a sincere appreciation for being able to be around for my children. I also knew, however, that if circumstances in my life hadn't allowed for that, somehow we would have figured it out just as my own mother had.

I was happy when the holidays arrived and we all went up to Sugarloaf in Maine for a week of skiing with some old friends. Erin was able to enter their ski-school program which I was comfortable with, although I noticed her limp had once again increased. Her life was jam-packed with events so I assumed the increased activity level was probably fatiguing her foot.

The skiing went fine for the kids, although the adults looked a bit frazzled after a week of ministering to six children. Soon it was home again, back to school, and a return to reality.

January is always special since it is the month of Erin's birth. How well I remember looking like a "weary watermelon" a month longer than I anticipated, since everything indicated Erin was to be born in December. This particular year, 1986, she decided on a swim party. Eight-year-olds are much like sea porpoises in the water: up and down, up and down, with lots of snorting, spitting, and coughing. After the party, as Kevin and I said good-bye to the last guest, I headed for the nearest chair and longed for "temporaries" to replace my very permanent and tired feet.

Life is curious. You think you're winning only to find out that once again, there's a glitch. That's the most accurate way I can describe Erin's life with congenital scoliosis. There was never any indication of why things changed; they simply did, and Erin, like many other scoliosis patients, had no choice but to reconcile herself. Over time we learned that some things might not be able to be corrected. Little by little, we came to the realization that there was a good chance her back would never be straight, but we continued to pray for a miracle.

I have learned a lot from Erin, most of which cannot be found in books. She was a remarkable child to live with because her insights about her birth defects were so mature and so accepting. Kevin finally was coming to the same realization as I: this was probably never going to end and I was delighted when, in February, he decided to join Erin and me for her appointment with Dr. Goldberg. Things didn't look so great to me and I thought it would be important for Kevin to hear firsthand how Erin's condition was progressing. Also, I looked forward to having a little more support there, not just for Erin, but for me as well.

We had a normal routine — check in, pull out hospital card, get parking ticket stamped, and then off to X ray. We knew everyone there and it was more like a social visit than a doctor's appointment. From radiology we entered the examining room and awaited the verdict. I remember the look on Kevin's face when he saw her first X ray in three years; it was never easy. I can only imagine what it was like for Erin.

Dr. Goldberg conducted a thorough examination and explained to us that she was in the midst of a growth spurt to which he attributed the increase in her curve. Medically, we would have to take one day at a time. He suggested we consider trying electrode stimulation but made no promises as to its success. Electrode stimulation (a device for applying electronic pulses) had been around for several years, but it had only recently received FDA approval. Generally, it was not used on children, especially if their spine had been fused. Since only five of Erin's vertebrae had been fused, Dr. Goldberg felt it was worth consideration since it would give Erin an opportunity to be out of her brace for the first time at night in many years.

The electrode stimulator itself resembled a walkman. The wires were inserted in two electrode patches placed on Erin's back a specified distance apart. When activated, the apparatus stimulated the muscle and created a force that pushed on the spine. If successful, the stimulation would prevent further curvature.

There were no guarantees as to its success or whether Erin could tolerate the unusual sensation the stimulator would create. The thought of another adjustment seemed unfair but if it could possibly help, it was worth a try. We left with Erin agreeing to try it if her case was approved. We explained to Erin that if she was very uncomfortable she could go right back to the body jacket. During the weeks we waited for the stimulator, Erin showed normal signs of concern, which I shared.

About two weeks later our call came and we were told someone named Tony would be flying up from New Jersey. March 14 was a dreary, rainy day, which ultimately delayed the flight. Tony was a warm, likable guy in his late twenties or early thirties who seemed to enjoy not only his role, but kids as well. He and Florence, the assistant, got to work immediately, measuring Erin's back to place the electrodes far enough apart to be effective. Due to Erin's fusions, they only had about five centimeters available with which to work. Erin's combination of birth defects forced them to place the electrodes in an unconventional spot, but one that would temporarily prove to be effective for her back.

It was clear to me that Erin might be getting into something perhaps more uncomfortable than the brace, although easier to wear. We would have to measure her back every few days to make sure we were placing the electrodes in the correct spot. Erin would need nearly an adult level of the stimulation to push her spine back. This was going to be an interesting time in her life.

Erin was doing fine until we got into the car after the appointment. Then she unloaded and I was relieved to see her let go. Not only did she cry, she became furious at me. That was a fairly memorable ride home and I'm sure the people who passed us wondered what I did to be so naughty. It was as if everything Erin had ever felt about her back was just rolling out — the longest run-on sentence in history. You know what, her reaction was normal and healthy, but the sad part was that there was nothing she said that I could possibly disagree with. She was absolutely correct. It wasn't fair.

When we got home, Erin stayed in the car. I guess she didn't like living with us that day. The boys were upset with me for leaving her there and I think they were also shocked to see their sister react this way. Colin, a real fan of machines, was frustrated because he wanted to see the new apparatus. I don't know how, but in his own special way he managed to get her out of the car, into the kitchen, and finally, even coaxed her in to giving a demonstration. Breen and Colin looked like two kids experimenting with a wonderful new gadget, which made Erin feel better about her new device.

There are ups and downs for everyone in life and although Erin was having more than her share, she plugged away in her usual amazing style. Feeling her own body twenty-four hours a day was special and she talked about how good that was. On March 27 we returned to the hospital to meet Tony again. Erin had done nicely with the stimulator so we agreed to purchase one. At the most, we hoped for six months of success, a long time in our scheme of things.

Erin continued plugging along. During this time she won third place in an essay contest on the topic "Why I Love America." Erin didn't just love America, she seemed to love life, and her appreciation for each day was a lesson for all of us. Lots of things and people were instrumental in helping Erin to develop this wonderful attitude. Her second-grade teacher, Miss O'Connell, played a big part. When we got our new puppy, Foolish, in we went, dog and all, for everyone to meet our "foolish" new pet. Miss O'Connell had even suggested that Erin bring in her stimulator for "show-and-tell." Can you imagine the look on the parents' faces at dinner that night when their little ones said, "Oh, Erin Mahony brought her stimulator in for show-and-tell today!" Also, the fact that Miss O'Connell was retiring after forty-four years of teaching brought with it lots of attention, parties, and even the press. There was no doubt in my mind that second grade would stand out as an exceptional year in Erin's history.

◌◦◌

The summer of 1986 turned out to be the most chaotic one we had spent since moving to our new home. Why anyone decides to do home remodeling is absolutely beyond me. We had a new puppy, no kitchen, and Kevin would leave me with long lists of instructions for the workmen and then dash off to his other life. I was surrounded by six men, kids who were tired of living in the rough by week two, a dog who constantly had to go for walks, more dirt than you could ever imagine, and Erin, who wandered around asking me to check to see if her stimulator was turned on. Picture it! To get to the basement we had to walk out the front door, around the house, and into another door. Our attire was something to see and in the midst of it all, Colin's friend Frieder arrived from Germany.

In July, Erin and I went off to Dr. Goldberg to see how the stimulator was doing; the verdict was not good. The measurement of her curve had increased 3° since April, but there was always a standard deviation, so we agreed to go three more months. We also stopped by for a visit with Dr. Scott since Erin had been having a lot of headaches. He gave her a thorough going over and felt that the source might be stress. Erin worried a lot about the success of the stimulator and I'm not sure she was as invested in it as we thought. But she was willing to do whatever we suggested to try to help her back.

⚭⚭

After the July visit I was feeling less positive. Erin was looking more and more tilted to me, and others were commenting as well. At times, the whole situation made me very sad, but I would pull myself out of that mood by thinking back to the day she was first diagnosed. Erin had come a long way. Her ability to deal with the ups and downs of her birth defects was amazing for everyone who met her, most especially for me. Like all mothers, I accepted the road Erin had to travel but I prayed that, at some future time, it would become a road less traveled for other children. The detours seemed to be ongoing and the work was simply never finished.

The summer seemed to fly by for the children, but our construction site appeared as if it was never going to end. In the midst of it all, unbeknownst to me, the cabinetmaker left for a three-week vacation. The man who was going to do our tiles needed knee surgery so the mystery of my walls piggybacked with the cabinetmaker's time off. When the cabinetmaker came back on the job, he shattered the door to my new stove the day he installed it. Fortunately, he wasn't seriously hurt, but the saga of a new door was yet to be solved. The next day the electrician walked through the screen in the atrium door that I had patiently awaited for six weeks, and that occurred after he misplaced the directions to our alarm system. For sure, no one was happier than I when September finally arrived and I would soon have a workable kitchen. In the end it was worth all the upheaval.

I should probably thank all of our workmen for the diversion since it really kept my mind off Erin. You can only imagine how excited our three children were when the first day of school came simply to know they would be in a building most of the day that had no plaster dust in it.

Erin began third grade with Mrs. Kehoe, a dynamic teacher; Colin entered seventh grade; and Breen was a freshman in high school. As for me, I was still finishing my CAES degree at Boston College and working as an aide in Erin's school. It didn't take long for people to notice Erin's limp had increased and that she appeared a bit more tilted. In the mornings she walked to school, but by afternoon she was pooped, and I would often give her a ride home. Sports had started once again and Erin returned to soccer, this time wearing her back brace, which troubled the soccer league. We sent off a letter waiving them of any liability and they were satisfied. Erin really loved the game. Some kids wore braces on their teeth, some wore glasses: Erin's brace was on her back. No big deal.

As the weeks passed, Erin formulated her own diagnosis and began commenting that the stimulator was not working. She was unhappy with her posture and could clearly see the change. "Mom, can they fix me?" she would ask. "Why is my back doing this?" was another favorite question. Her tummy was beginning to protrude a bit because of the lordosis caused by her fusions.

On November 17 it was time to return to Dr. Goldberg. I was pretty sure that this was not going to be a good visit and Erin felt the same. As soon as Florence saw the X rays, it was obvious to her that the electrodes were no longer in the right location, in spite of our measuring. Poor Dr. Goldberg arrived at what must have appeared a most unhappy gathering. He immediately measured the X rays to get a degree reading of Erin's curvature. As he proceeded, Florence shared her news about the electrodes.

Dr. Goldberg had a style all his own and often, in the midst of a crisis, he would very casually mention a new course of action as if it had been on the back burner of his brain all the time. I'm sure it had. He agreed that the curve was unquestionably worse and felt that he needed another set of X rays before making a decision. He suggested that we return to radiology and then break for lunch.

Kevin went back to his office and Erin and I returned to our old friends in radiology. While we waited, she talked about the stimulator: she was disappointed that it wasn't working and that things were getting worse, but she hated my ripping the tape off her back every morning. Erin's skin was very sensitive despite our using non-allergenic tape. We were both happy that at least we had tried.

After we finished in X ray, we delivered the pictures to Dr. Goldberg's office and set off to the snack bar for lunch. I could see that Erin was worried. We were both anxious to get back and hear the latest solution. On this occasion Dr. Goldberg began by diagramming two spines. The first was what he had hoped Erin's spine would do, but did not. The second was the path Erin's spine had taken. As I glanced over I saw that Erin's face was absolutely expressionless as she perused an X ray of her back that indicated a very significant curve. As I shifted my attention back to Dr. Goldberg, he was explaining that if Erin wore a back brace twenty-two hours a day, it might counteract the curve. This time he suggested a Milwaukee brace. Knowing how devastated Erin would be wearing this model to school, he agreed to allow her to keep her body jacket on at school and put a Milwaukee brace on at home from three in the afternoon until the next morning. We had finally hit the jackpot — big-time baggage.

The Milwaukee brace was very different from the others. It was the one item Erin had hoped she would never have to model. The Milwaukee was made of bars attached to a neck piece that stretched the spine and placed the chin in an almost exaggerated pose. Dr. Goldberg was trying to avoid surgery so that Erin could continue developing. Once fused, those vertebrae do not grow and she already had had five fused as a toddler. I could now see the light and realized that the real challenge for Erin was far into the future.

We always tried to find a little good news and this particular time it meant that for three weeks Erin could go without wearing anything on her body since it would take that long for this new brace to be made. For her that was better than a new bike: to simply go to bed and wake up each morning in her very own body.

I recall three very troubling weeks. Erin worried about the possibility of further surgery, alluded to by Dr. Goldberg as a possibility at some point not that far into the future. He had some concerns about where things were going and so did I. But Erin had the ability to really "zing" it out and the questions she posed were absolutely remarkable for her age. One day she asked me to put myself in her position and brainstorm how I could make it better for myself. Rather unprepared for the question, I looked at her for a few minutes and then said, "Erin, I think I would hope to do it the same way you are, taking one day at a time." Perhaps not the answer she expected but surely the best I could give.

Erin always bounced these visits off the boys, who each had his own way of processing and reacting to any new information. When she told Colin there was a possibility of another operation, he ended up picking on her for some foolish thing and stormed up the stairs. This was most unusual behavior. He hated hospitals but more than that he hated it when I wasn't around. Next came Breen. Erin passed on the possibility of more surgery and shared with Breen that she would have to wear back braces most of the time. "Oh great," Breen replied, "they don't need to operate. That means Dad can buy some magazine subscriptions from me." He was selling them as a fund-raiser for his class, and I think both Erin and I were so shocked by his reaction that we ended up in a fit of laughter. As long as Erin had brothers she would never become a little princess.

I spent the ensuing weeks talking to Erin's school principal, nurse, and teacher preparing them for the new package. They were extremely supportive and the school nurse even went into Erin's class and did a presentation on braces and scoliosis. It answered a lot of questions for Erin's peers and made Erin feel a lot more comfortable.

In the midst of all this Erin decided she wanted to learn how to ice skate, so off we went for skates. Fitting her left foot was a real challenge. The class skating party was a big deal for Erin and for me, nearly the cause of an ulcer. In order to realize Erin's wish, I was to be the "support" and Erin the "skater." Holding Erin up was hard since I weighed about 110 pounds and she was at least half of that. I hadn't skated in years; it was quite a show. When we got home, it was clear just by looking at Erin that this would not be one of her better sports, nor mine. But at least we had tried.

∞∞

Erin became more and more anxious about her new brace and along with her anxiety came headaches. At first, I didn't make the connection, but the closer we came to the day, the worse the headaches became. Certainly, she had been on a roller coaster for a long time and I wasn't at all surprised at her reaction.

On December 9 we were off to the hospital. Erin loved school and insisted on attending the first hour and a half of her day. When we arrived at the Floating, the orthotist had only one of Erin's braces ready, which softened the blow a bit. Her day brace would not be much different from what she had been wearing each night. Erin quickly took note of the new modifications, so I simply kept my comments to myself and let the orthotist take over. He was absolutely wonderful. Unfortunately, there were some differences that would be major to Erin: for one, she would not be able to reach down and attend to her shoes. She was so annoyed about this that she found a way to lie down on the floor to get them on. Finally, we prevailed upon her to go model her new brace for Dr. Goldberg so he could check out how it fit and suggest any necessary adjustments.

I am convinced that the only way children survive these experiences is by finding a doctor who is perceptive enough to allow them to vent their frustrations. It was clear to Dr. Goldberg that Erin was quite annoyed and uncomfortable. He immediately changed hats and allowed her to spew, listening to her every word. Much to Erin's surprise, Dr. Goldberg agreed with everything she said. "Young lady," he said, "you are absolutely right, but I think if you give this a few weeks, it will give you some relief and you will eventually feel better with it on." Erin wasn't completely sold on the idea but we had two more weeks before the Milwaukee would be ready so it would give us time to adjust to this one.

The next few weeks were tough and I spent most of my time trying to help Erin deal with the pressure sores that came from having a brace on twenty-two hours a day. The school nurse was helpful and removed it for about an hour each morning. The nights were difficult: Erin would wake up and have difficulty getting back to sleep, probably due to the anticipation of yet another brace. But she always had a great line. She'd tiptoe in and suddenly I'd hear this little voice say, "Mom, are you busy?" When we got desperate, I'd take the brace off for forty-five minutes, set the alarm, and let her sleep unencumbered. Somehow she thought that was a great compromise and would get back to sleep after the "free time." How she managed to get herself off to school in the morning used to amaze me.

The boys found all this very confusing. They really weren't big enough to understand that Erin's scoliosis was not going to go away and that there were some things that doctors couldn't fix. I explained to them that the doctors needed money to fund research into looking for ways to alleviate this condition. Suddenly a light went off in my own head and I realized that it was perhaps time to begin the "Erin Mahony Scoliosis Research Fund." Although the kitty would be a drop in the bucket, in time it would grow and make a dent in an area that affects an incredible number of children each year. Today that fund is available to provide research opportunities for those interested in helping children like Erin who long to have a "straighter" future.

∽∾

Suddenly, it was December 23, and while the rest of the world was preparing for the holidays, Erin and I were on our way to the Floating to see her "Mercedes-Benz" of braces. The unveiling of this well-known model was a time of quiet emotions for us both. I was impressed by its openness, but the neck piece was an amazing sight. In addition to that modification, it also had two straps that went under each arm. When I looked at it as an alternative to surgery, the craftsmanship was mind-boggling and most impressive.

Dr. Goldberg easily could have had another career in sales. He worked overtime with Erin convincing her that this was the way to go. Erin's only concern was the neck and chin modification, which finally made her wearing of a brace most apparent. It was clear that I needed to find a vehicle to convince Erin that "who she was" had nothing to do with her condition. It was her qualities as a human being and how she chose to live her life that really counted. Such an easy statement for an observer to make. In time, Erin came to understand all this but at that particular moment it certainly wasn't a priority.

I gave Erin the space she needed to adjust but I really blew it at dinner that first night by serving one of her favorites, tacos, which she couldn't even see. The neck piece took some adjusting to and the engineering of it made eating a less enjoyable experience. No one warns you of these things because they haven't had the experience themselves. Erin's first "Milwaukee meal" was quite a show. The condiments were spilling everywhere and Kevin and the boys were speechless. Even the dog hesitated to go for the scraps.

Later, I made the mistake of suggesting that dinner be a brace-free time as Erin was attempting to get into her pajama bottoms. She couldn't bend over to see what she was doing with them, either. I'm sure she wanted to wring my neck. After I helped her get them on, which also injured her pride, she looked at me and said a very curt "good night." That was my cue to leave.

I often used my walks with our dog Foolish as "think" time and on that particular evening I was wondering how I would ever manage to make this transition a smoother one for Erin. I realized it was a time that she needed to work out for herself and my job was merely to be the supportive bystander.

⌘

January and February of 1987 were crisis months for Erin: nausea in the morning, followed by a breakfast of Coca-Cola and crackers at ten o'clock in school. We camouflaged the soda in a thermos and her teacher, Mrs. Kehoe, won a gold star for nursing skills, which she almost packed in on one particular morning when Erin literally "lost her crackers" all over her desk. That was a real test of the durability of the classroom teacher and a clue to me that it was time to address this condition. Dr. Goldberg felt Erin's reflux problem had returned and I was hoping it was simply for a short visit.

On February 12, my thirty-ninth birthday, Erin and I ended up spending most of that day and a good part of the evening at the Floating with Dr. Harris, head of pediatric surgery. The grand finale of the visit was an upper G.I. series for Erin. She downed the barium swallow as if it were a milkshake and I recalled the same behavior she had shown at the age of nine months. We left soon after and awaited the results at home since the boys were anxiously looking forward to my birthday dinner, a phone call away to the Chinese Gourmet. Kevin was off in Florida, missing my birthday for the first time in eighteen years. But, as always, the troops made it extra special and it ended up being a very short but very memorable day.

That wonderful, accommodating service which we were so used to at the Floating hadn't changed one bit and by nine o'clock I was on the phone with Dr. Harris. The film showed that Erin had a slight kink in her esophagus but he was of the opinion that the nausea was due to all the emotional ups and downs she had had to deal with, especially those caused by the neck apparatus on her brace. Just to be sure, we then moved on to a gastroenterologist. Dr. Thompson, a quiet and gentle man, felt that Erin had no blockage and that we should continue with Pepto-Bismol as well as some good family support. It was time for everyone to accept Erin's birth defects and to understand that they were not going to disappear and might get worse before they got better, if they got better.

∞∞

The rest of Erin's third-grade year shifted its focus to the cast of characters she knew as her family. Erin hated the Milwaukee, but freely admitted that it did make her more comfortable and most of all, a lot straighter. The boys made a concerted effort to communicate how they felt about all this, and Erin, being the wonderful listener that she is, accepted their feelings but not without adding a few of her own. That was fair play.

Before we knew it Erin and the boys were once again out on the soccer field. It was summer and everyone was involved in their respective interests. I spent my free time going to graduate school and putting the finishing touches on my coursework so that I could student teach in the fall. Dr. Goldberg continued to see Erin regularly and said that all we could do was wait and hope that time would be on her side. With Erin still in a growth spurt, we went back and forth to the Floating for adjustments to keep up with the contour of her ever-changing body. Within the Milwaukee apparatus, things seemed to be relatively stable.

It was at this point that I stopped writing in the journal and so I am relying on a few notes here and there, but predominantly on her medical reports. I'm not sure what made me finally stop. For me, writing was as flexible as it was permanent, and even though I wanted to believe that in my writing about Erin there was still hope for change and improvement, in my heart I felt that her curvature had become as enduring as the thoughts I penned. I had spent a great deal of time helping Erin to deal with her congenital scoliosis. And yet, when asked what it was and how she got it, I still found myself stumbling through the explanation. The definition of this birth defect seemed to be changing all the time. I knew the ways in which it had complicated Erin's life, but in the quiet of a moment, I still didn't understand exactly what it meant in terms of the future. Like many children with birth defects, Erin is unique and so I'm not so sure anyone could look into a crystal ball and say "This is where Erin will be ten years from now." It was really time for me to step back from all this and immerse myself into something that offered greater certainty.

CHAPTER TWELVE
Prelude

A s Breen moved into his sophomore year of high school, Colin into his eighth-grade year in middle school, and Erin into fourth grade, I began my student teaching, something that I had hoped to do some ten years earlier. It was clear that circumstances had caused me to grow in many ways that I'm not sure would have happened without Erin's birth defects. I felt confident that I would have a lot to offer as a special-education teacher.

Erin's situation remained unchanged and in the fall of 1987 spinal studies were done upon the suggestion of Drs. Goldberg and Scott, just to be sure nothing was going on that we were unaware of. It revealed no significant changes.

The following January, 1988, it was clear that the Milwaukee was still holding Erin's curve at 35°. But when she was out of it for prolonged periods of time, the discomfort was most apparent. She had been given an exercise program to follow on a regular basis, but she was going through one of those spells in which she felt that the pressures on her were getting out of control. Erin had never really known the luxury of a life without structure.

Fourth grade was an academically successful year for Erin. Her teacher, Mrs. Gay, provided her with a wonderful reading program as well as many other exciting forms of enrichment. In spite of all the interruptions that life brings with it, I successfully completed my practicums and was preparing to take my comps for graduate school. While I was quietly thrilled with the near-completion of my dream, to the troops it was merely a question of "When can we start having homemade desserts again?" Breen had just turned sixteen years old and I will never forget how weird it felt when he drove me to the store. That was a very exciting time in his life and for me as his mom, a clue that he was now quite the young man.

⌒⌒

Late in the summer of 1988, just before school began, Erin visited Dr. Goldberg. Within a period of about three months her back had gone from a 35° curve to one of 43°. Her scoliosis was showing the early signs of slumping. The growth spurt was continuing to maintain itself in the same controlling fashion as before. This was not good news. Dr. Goldberg knew that Erin did not like wearing the Milwaukee to school but he truly felt that it would be the best solution to control the increasing curve. It wouldn't solve what was already there, but it would serve as a stronger force than the Boston brace.

Erin had actually been wearing the Milwaukee all summer with the exception of when she was swimming or participating in sports. Dr. Goldberg had seen what was coming and presented such a good rationale behind his efforts to find solutions to these changes that Erin would eventually comply. As she got older, it was clear to me that he really held all the cards in terms of her level of cooperation. He empowered her to make her own decisions and because of this, Erin was able to relate to her back in a reasonable way.

⌒⌒

The complexities of Erin's transition to the Milwaukee were soon balanced by a new man in her life, Paul Joyce, her fifth-grade teacher. Paul had also taught Colin and so he knew our family very well. An outstanding human being, he made Erin's fifth-grade experience one she would never forget. She had a portfolio of Mr. Joyce stories, which she always shared at dinner.

The highlight of being a fifth-grader in Erin's school is a week-long ecology trip. Since she was not able to get in and out of her brace on her own, roommates played a key role in the success of ventures such as these. She had been fortunate to have had a fantastic group of friends who all knew the secrets to getting the brace comfortably in position on Erin's body. She used to tell me that some of them were better at it than I was and no doubt that was probably true. The fifth-grade teachers, most of whom were women, agreed to pitch in whenever Erin needed help. They were outstanding and assured me that all would be fine. When departure time came, I don't think I ever saw anyone as excited as Erin was to get on that bus and go off to Camp Grotonwood. She certainly had no problem separating and was quite the traveler.

As a fifth-grader she also enjoyed being the crossing guard for the kindergartners. Erin absolutely adored these little ones and I remember one in particular who had a mad crush on her. I think at one point he may have even given her a kiss on the cheek. Developmentally, this was truly one of Erin's very best years and it was clear to me that she could easily take care of herself. The only accommodation was an extra set of books for home since carrying a heavy book bag was difficult.

Erin's life at this time was medically uneventful. Her gait had improved and her nausea, while never completely gone, seemed to be under control. Things had essentially stabilized. The boys were doing fine and each had found an interest that made school not only enjoyable, but an enriching experience. Before we knew it, summer had arrived. That summer, in particular, seemed to just zoom by. Erin attended a day camp for about six weeks and spent the rest of the summer focusing on her tennis. By the end, she had become quite proficient.

∽∾

As I looked to the fall, I knew that middle school would be an adjustment for Erin. She was still sporting the Milwaukee brace and there would be students there from three other schools in town, many of whom did not know her and what this was all about. The curiosity factor is there for all of us and Erin was always very perceptive about changes and how they translated for her. Despite all this, she made the transition beautifully.

I had always walked my kids to school on the first day. It was a tradition, after pictures and a few good hugs. The week before school began Erin really vacillated as to whether or not it would be appropriate for me to walk her. Now I realize that hurting my feelings was the issue here and that she really didn't need my company anymore. When the time arrived she allowed me to walk her to the corner but no hugs or kisses on the street. I laughed and thanked her for allowing me to accompany her at all. Well, we proceeded to the end of our street and then up the next a bit. Erin stopped, looked at me and said, "Okay, that's as far as you can go, Mom. Now please, no big good-byes; just go home and thanks!" That was the very last time I ever walked any of my kids to school.

I had already sent a note off to all of Erin's teachers asking for extra copies of the textbooks for home and apprising them of her situation. They just needed to know about her brace and a few limitations in gym. Communication with teachers is important. Rather than physically appearing at school, which is really a "no-no" from your child's perspective, a simple note at the beginning of the year answers any questions.

Erin had an absolutely wonderful year and the grand finale was a trip to Maryland to participate in National History Day. She and four other students had written a play about inventions which had won in the regionals, continued on to the states, and suddenly, we were on a bus on our way to the University of Maryland for the nationals. Marie Doyle, Erin's social studies teacher, had been a true inspiration to these students and look at what had unfolded for them as a result of all her energy and enthusiasm. On June 12 we loaded a bus-full of kids from all over Massachusetts and set off to Maryland. Four days later I stood proudly in the arena of the University of Maryland as our little Belmont sixth-graders, serenaded by the U.S. Navy Band, received third place. It was one of the proudest moments of my life. What a fabulous way to end your first year of middle school.

∞∞

The summer between sixth and seventh grades was enriched by new experiences for Erin, highlighted by her first stay at overnight camp. On the recommendation of one of Erin's friends, we had chosen Camp Hayward, a YMCA facility. I had called the camp earlier in the spring and explained that other than the extra appendage of the brace, Erin was a normal, enthusiastic, wonderful kid and would be an easy camper. I made a special request and asked if Erin's good friend, Emily Cook, could be her bunkmate. Erin was unable to get the brace on and off herself and also needed help with her physical therapy. Emily was a great friend and had gained a clear understanding of what it was like not to have life just the way you might have expected it to be. Since this would also be Emily's first year there, it made sense for them to bunk together. And that's exactly what they did.

Erin's choices for activities at camp did have some limitations: no gymnastics, no horseback riding, no water skiing. But she was able to live vicariously through the experiences of her friends and at no time in her life has she ever harbored any resentment. Surely, a little longing, but no resentment.

Erin's camp experience was the highlight of her summer and the topper was leaving with the honorary camper pin for her unit. That was a wonderful summer for the boys as well. Breen graduated from high school in June, having been a co-captain of the swim team his senior year, and spent the summer as a lifeguard at a private club. Colin was mowing a few lawns with his good friend Ben and anxiously awaiting his sixteenth birthday.

As Erin prepared to begin seventh grade at the middle school and Colin looked forward to his junior year in high school, Breen was getting ready to leave for his freshman year at Lehigh University in Bethlehem, Pennsylvania. The adjustment was a difficult one for me since Breen had been the one I depended on to fix and assemble things and close up at night when Kevin traveled. Like me, he was a night owl, and I knew that I would miss his company.

Erin and Colin were also sad about Breen's leaving, especially Colin. The boys had shared the third floor of our house for several years and they were very close. They had experienced a lot together, including the time Kevin and I entertained guests in the living room as firecrackers came exploding out our third-floor windows. Creativity remains one of their strong points.

Before we knew it, we were a house of four, plus Foolish, and school was back in session, not just for the children but for me as well. I had finally realized my dream and taken on a job at the children's former grammar school as a part-time resource teacher. It was a big decision, but it was really time for me to do my thing. For the most part everyone was supportive.

∞∞

As Erin prepared for the first day of seventh grade, it was clear to me that the little girl was gone and I was in the company of a very attractive pre-adolescent. Clothes shopping took on a whole new tone as my opinions were no longer valid and I found myself wandering aimlessly in stores searching for a bench for my very weary legs. The end result was never more than a few outfits; the challenge was fitting Erin's body, whose contours were quite different from those of others her age. As much as I loathed these long expeditions, I learned to keep my comments to myself since I could only imagine how disappointing it must have been for Erin. She was never able to wear what she really wanted. Manny, our tailor, who had assumed an important part in Erin's daily existence, was always willing to do an instant rebirth of a pair of jeans or a skirt. Hemming was also a challenge since Erin's curving had created a crease to one side. These were all the tricks I learned along the way. I ached for the families who could not afford these options.

Basically, we had to invest in two wardrobes, which needed replenishing each time the brace had major alterations. We had the "in-brace" outfits and the "out-brace" outfits; both shared equal importance. Erin was meticulous about her person, but that was not hard to understand either. She had an appreciation and respect for her body that far surpassed most people's. Most important, she had a sensitivity to people that someone else might not even consider. Erin had learned early on what it was like to deal with differences.

Erin enjoyed seventh grade. She loved learning and was an excellent student. Most of all, she delighted in her friends, and so did we. Physically,

Erin was getting some unexpected and very painful muscle spasms. They often took her off guard and all she could do was wait them out. Exercising and using the physical therapy program she had been taught was the key to avoiding a muscle spasm; but this particular fall that was not working so well. Her body looked almost as if it had "rotated" to me but having never experienced any of this before, I couldn't be sure. I knew something was different because Erin seemed uncomfortable in her brace.

On December 21, once again, while the rest of the world prepared for the arrival of Santa Claus, there we were, getting Erin fitted with a new brace, a redesign of an old model. We had gone to see Dr. Goldberg in early December and he confirmed my suspicions that we were once again in another growth spurt, but this time something new had been added, "rotation." If Erin was standing still looking at me, one shoulder leaned back and off in a different direction. The image is hard to explain but it was not good news and it could not be completely corrected surgically. As the spine was twisting on its axis, it not only distorted Erin's ribs, but, in fact, was rotating her entire body. This was something I had read about years earlier, never dreaming that Erin would become one of those statistics.

The new brace had chunks of padding in areas that were very uncomfortable for Erin. The one outstanding characteristic was that it no longer had the neck piece and had departed from the design of the Milwaukee, taking on the ostensible appearance of a much-modified Boston brace. Erin's curve was at about 43°, so it was important that she wear this new brace faithfully. The adjustment would not be an easy one and Erin felt very uncomfortable.

To address her muscle spasms, a new physical therapist prescribed a program quite different from the previous one. More and more physical therapy had become the key not only to comfort, but to appearance as well, as it kept Erin's tummy trim so that the scoliosis would not develop into a pronounced kyphosis or protruding stomach. It was at this point that Erin and I both realized the physical therapy or an exercise program for her back might be part of her agenda for life.

We spent our winter holiday vacation relaxing in Vermont and in early January we returned to Dr. Goldberg for a brace check. In general Erin was adjusting nicely to her new device due in part to the creation of a new undershirt for sensitive skin. Invented by a company out in the Midwest, the new shirt was fashioned of a fabric similar to chamois cloth. It was seamless and remained in place under the brace. As a result, Erin had no brace rubs and was thrilled that once again, another door had opened. The design of the brace held her nicely, even without the superstructure of the neck piece. You can only imagine how exciting this new model was for Erin since she could camouflage it somewhat under her clothing. Nothing protruded so that it was not obvious to the observer that she had this extra piece of baggage. Keeping in mind that Erin was now almost an adolescent, this was an important improvement for her. It meant that people would no longer give that second look, wondering why such a pretty young lady was in such a piece of equipment.

Academically, seventh grade moved along very nicely for Erin and I think the highlight of that year was making the middle school basketball team. She shared a jersey but was thrilled to be playing a game which she not only loved, but had mastered. She had come a long way and with a lot of perseverance had become a fairly decent athlete.

We finished up the year, visited Dr. Goldberg for an X ray and brace check, and began the summer stretch. Erin talked more and more about the day when she could get rid of her brace and often asked me how much more I thought she would grow. Her goal was to be at least five feet tall and she was almost there. She vacillated about the possibility of more surgery and, I'm sure, fantasized about being straight like everyone else.

∞∞

During the summer between seventh and eighth grades, Erin did her traditional activities — two weeks at Camp Hayward, a week at Bentley College basketball camp, and overnights with good friends. The boys were both working — Breen as a waiter and Colin mowing lawns. I suggested a summer vacation, which no one seemed to welcome, so I proposed to Erin that we go by ourselves. It was the two hundredth anniversary of Mozart's death and so we set off for ten days in Austria and Germany.

Traveling on planes was an uncomfortable experience for Erin. Wearing a brace and sitting in those movie-theater type seats is not easy for anyone. This particular trip left her unusually uncomfortable and even after a good day's rest in the hotel, we paced our exploring and often took cabs for short jaunts. Having her all to myself for almost two weeks made me increasingly aware of how she had deteriorated and was really slowing down. But Erin was wonderful company and it really wouldn't have mattered where we went, it was simply nice to be together. I remember feeling that same way when I had the boys alone. That was really prime time, when you had one of your children all to yourself. They actually talked to you in full sentences, sometimes even paragraphs! A parent's dream.

While I was enjoying having Erin all to myself, Kevin was also having fun with the boys. I can only imagine what the house looked like and what they ate for dinner. Domestic skills were not Kevin's forte. Fortunately for him, the boys were a bit stronger in that area.

Erin and I had a wonderful time and we talked about everything and anything. We got ripped off at amusement parks, shopped until our toes felt like they were leaving our feet, and our favorite thing of all, feasted on Sacher torte at Demel's in Vienna. In the quiet of a moment, we sometimes talked about Erin's perception of her birth defect, which was simply that you accept the things you cannot change. Although she talked about how lucky she felt that it wasn't anything worse than congenital scoliosis and was almost convincing, it was clear to me that her concern about her appearance was growing. A few times she let her guard down and hinted at how wonderful it would be if someone could make it all better. But she was pretty sure that would never happen.

When we got back from Europe, it was once again time for school to begin. Breen set off for his sophomore year at Lehigh and Colin was beginning his senior year in high school. Colin had masterfully taken over Breen's role as my backup and he had become my buddy. He was my fix-it person, the audiovisual king, the guardian of the dog, and most of all, a fantastic human being to be around, most of the time. Breen's stepping out of the picture gave Colin the space to be his own person, which so often happens when the dynamics of a family change. In addition to all these things, Colin was as good at acting as Breen was at drawing. I was a very lucky mother and I thrived on watching all our children as they participated in their various interests. And Kevin readjusted his work schedule and was spending more time at home. He was learning that the experiences you have with children are once-in-a-lifetime.

⚭

Since eighth grade is a stepping-stone to high school, you can only imagine how exciting that first day of school was for Erin. I found it extremely hard to believe that Colin was now in his last year of high school, and even though he hoped the year would fly by, I wanted it to go on forever, at least the good parts. The stress of the college application process I could have lived without, but then again, just think of how Colin felt. This period of development is often a test of wills, "Will I win or will she?" It was almost impossible ever to get angry at Colin because he would look at you with this blank stare, change his voice to that of someone much older, look you straight in the eye and say, "Now Mary, do you really feel that way about this? Come on now Mary, take a chill pill!" Breen had a more direct approach when we disagreed. "Mom, you need to get a life," he would say. The spontaneity was a nice touch, but there were times I could have lived without it. In spite of these moments, having both of them away would be a real adjustment for all of us. Ours would be a much quieter house.

Erin had no sooner begun school than it was once again time for a trip to Dr. Goldberg. She now got pretty anxious before those visits and sometimes even broke out with eczema. Her sleep was uneven and she worried, as any of us would, because there was so much uncertainty as to whether she would be having another operation or living with what was clearly becoming a more severe curve. These were new clues as to how she was doing and they worried me.

When we were in Europe I noticed that her left foot seemed to tire easily. I'm not sure if it was the crease of her curve or the weakness in her foot, but there were times when she looked even more tilted. It wasn't just me; Erin noticed it as well and when she asked me about it, since I have never lied to her, I conceded that yes, I wondered the same thing. The lordosis or dip in the small of her back was the most bothersome to her. This was the one area she hoped a doctor could fix, since most of her muscle spasms occurred there. In spite of all her exercises, the spasms continued, but with much less frequency when she did her physical therapy program. Erin would lie down and I would massage the area until finally either the spasm quit or my fingers gave up.

Things were relatively unchanged in that September 1991 visit; oh, perhaps there was a slight increase to the curve but all in all, there was nothing remarkable. Erin talked freely to Dr. Goldberg. He made no promises as to what could be accomplished in surgery, but agreed that some correction could be done. Erin wanted to know, "How much longer will this curving continue?" the question that many children with scoliosis often ask. "You have about one year left of growth after menstruation" was his programmed response.

Erin's eighth grade seemed to fly by and like her other years, was a very successful one. Colin's senior year did not pass quite so smoothly as Erin's. Early on he developed a pilonidal cyst, a nasty little thing which was operated on in early December. Just when we thought Colin was all better, he came down with mononucleosis, not unusual for a high school senior who was burning the candle at both ends. Keeping Colin down was an exasperating experience, but he recovered and I think I did too. In many ways, it was nice to have the opportunity to be there for him as I had been for Erin.

CHAPTER THIRTEEN
It's Time

∽

S hortly before Erin completed eighth grade, she once again saw Dr. Goldberg. It was at this time that I realized that I needed to resume my writing and try to make some sense out of the book that I had begun so long before. The first several pages had been jotted in a spiral binder I had started it for Erin and the boys. It was my hope that it might serve as a resource to parents of all children with birth defects, most especially parents of children with scoliosis. The lack of information for the lay person always astonished me, it being a condition that strikes such large numbers of children. It was, and still is, my hope that this can also be used as a resource for physicians, not for the medical text, which is minimal, but in terms of how a doctor views a patient. Finally, I enjoy writing and find it to be a sort of catharsis to a long and incredible journey. Surely, this would be true for other parents as well.

On June 3, 1991, Dr. Goldberg discussed the risks of further surgery to Erin. Yes, they could do a cosmetic correction to her drooping shoulder, but the gamble involved in correcting some of her spinal issues was irreversible paralysis. Two operations would be required to accomplish everything. If the first was successful, Erin would still have to face the risks involved with the second procedure. At the time the possibility of paralysis was a bit overwhelming for any of us to consider pursuing this route. Although on the surface Erin seemed satisfied with what was a joint decision, this was not the case at all. It was what Erin thought she should do. It was what she thought we wanted her to do. Unfortunately, I wasn't perceptive enough to read between the lines until several months later.

Before long we had to go to Boston's Children's Hospital to see Dr. Scott for the annual checkup. He had moved his practice there a few years earlier. Like many families of children with birth defects, we were and still are scattered all over in terms of which hospital we go to for Erin's various medical needs.

Dr. Scott hadn't seen us for about two years, which was my oversight. Hard as I tried to cover all the bases, this was one time I had slipped up in the schedule, the end result being this hiatus. When Dr. Scott was on staff at the Floating, his office was located off the beaten track, and his patients had to follow the broken line to the elevator and take it up to his floor. Although there was no broken line to follow at Children's, I chuckled to myself each time we went to his office because the route to it was very much off the beaten track there as well, and again, his space left a lot to be desired.

No matter how much time passed between our visits, Dr. Scott always greeted us with a warm and heartfelt welcome. As was his pattern, he would address Erin directly and ask for an update: how were things going, how was she feeling, etc. I continued to take notes on her progress and would sometimes share my perspective as well. It was not unusual for Erin to correct me, an ongoing reminder that she was very much in control of her own life. At this particular visit, Erin explained that she was getting headaches, some nausea, and a tingling feeling in her upper thighs. We had shared this with Dr. Goldberg in June and he had encouraged us to move on to Dr. Scott to see if all was well in terms of her neurological issues. After a thorough examination, Dr. Scott suggested that we have an MRI done just to be sure all was secure, since he had some concerns about the deficit in her lower extremities as well as the possibility of retethering. Erin had not had a complete series of pictures since 1987. Anticipating that she might need an MRI (magnetic resonance imaging), Dr. Goldberg assured us that he would make the necessary arrangements to have the studies done at the Floating since this was a familiar environment. The start of school was on the horizon and we needed the results as soon as possible just in case the images indicated a need for further surgery.

Before we knew it, Erin was in a dressing room preparing for her MRI. Her anxiety over her body had escalated a bit. She was unfamiliar with the imaging technique and full of questions. Prior to the arrival of this machine, I had attended a meeting for volunteers at the Floating in regard to this new state-of-the-art modality. I was relieved that there was no radiation, since Erin had certainly had her fair share of X rays. With scoliosis you don't have many options if you want to follow the progression of the curve.

In terms of engineering, the whole MRI procedure is rather benign. You lie on a table in a room specially built for this machine and your head and upper body are electronically moved into a cylinder or tube. If you have claustrophobia, you might have a problem with this part of the procedure. Basically, you simply lie still while a machine takes a magnetic photo of the designated area of your body. The staff that is manning the controls is in another room and they talk to you through an intercom system. Erin reported that all you feel is a tingling sensation as the picture is being taken.

Our appointment happened to be in the evening, which suited Erin just fine. Since she was able to keep her body fairly still, there was no need to medicate her. It is important that you do not move during the filming so that they can achieve a clear picture. The whole process moved along rather quickly and, before we knew it, we were done and Erin was in the dressing room changing back into her clothes. Unfortunately, they called us a few days later and suggested that we repeat the imaging. At some point during the first procedure Erin must have taken a sudden breath, which created a very shadowy picture. She was not at all pleased about the inconvenience of going back, but it was in her own best interest to do so.

The second set of MRIs came out fine, but still Erin's doctors felt that they needed further views since there was a question about one specific area. You certainly do not want to operate on anyone unless you are absolutely sure there is a need to do so. Once again, we headed back. Erin was pretty adamant that she would not submit to a fourth visit. In my heart I knew that if we really needed another, like it or not, she would comply.

The retakes put us a bit behind schedule in terms of the start of school and the resolution as to whether or not Erin needed further surgery. This was hard for her, and it put a bit of a damper on what is usually an especially exciting transition, the start of high school. In order to expedite the situation, I volunteered to drive the MRIs over to Dr. Scott at Children's so that he could give us his answer without delay. He was more than willing to put some time aside and read them while I waited. After a short while he came out and announced that he felt there was no indication of retethering. He invited me in so that he could explain the area in question. It was clear that Dr. Scott had not expected to see such a progression in Erin's curve and was truly saddened by its advancing state. Looking at the images was especially overpowering for me. The distortion of her body was getting more and more pronounced, and it hurt me to even consider what it might be like if this progression continued. Although I should have left Dr. Scott's office rejoicing that further neurosurgery was not necessary, I left with a very heavy heart.

Once I got through the usual hospital traffic, I headed for home and I think I replayed Erin's MRIs over and over again in my mind. I thought back to how thrilled we were after the very first operation when Dr. Goldberg and Dr. Scott had done a yeoman's job of dealing with her diastematomyelia as well as all the hemivertebrae. Her curve had been brought back to approximately 27°. Then there was the second procedure, not as serious as the first, but complicated by Erin's spinal leak. Then all the braces and the constant exercising as well as the brief stint with electrode stimulation. Never did I appreciate the complexity of the spine and the central nervous system until we found out what it was like when things weren't working correctly. Scoliosis is such a sneaky condition.

As I pulled into my driveway I was quite aware that I was bringing two messages: "Super news, you don't need surgery," and "It's clear by your MRIs that your curve is still progressing and we'll just have to monitor it carefully and see what happens." After speaking with many other families of patients with scoliosis, I have learned that this scenario is a familiar one. At an age when the body is so important, this is not an easy load for any kid to bear. I could see that Erin was masking much of what she really felt.

As was so often the case, she focused on the news of no surgery and seemed quite relieved. Kevin shared this feeling as well, and I went off to bed that night feeling guilty that I was totally preoccupied with the images I had seen. My mind felt like the lens of a video camera, and I went back and forth over each picture until I could no longer focus and finally fell asleep.

∞∞

Erin loved high school and had absolutely no problem handling the work. She decided to pass on a fall sport, a great relief to me. Although she missed the team spirit and the excitement of competing, she was comfortable with her decision. At the end of her school day, she looked exhausted and would often take a nap. If I even hinted at the fact that she appeared to tire more easily, I was ostracized from any further conversation for the rest of the afternoon. Her nausea and headaches continued to surface, and I was convinced that her tilting body was a lot more work for her to tolerate than she would ever admit.

As the winter basketball season approached, Erin was out in the driveway perfecting her shooting and dribbling skills almost on a daily basis. She even tried jogging but her left leg was not very cooperative and she was totally winded. Perhaps it was merely her lack of conditioning, perhaps her changing body. I really don't know. On the basketball court, what Erin lacked in speed she often made up for in accuracy. She was delighted to see that she had survived the cut and made the junior varsity team. Although I talked to her coach on the phone and tried to explain that Erin had some neurological issues on her left side in addition to the scoliosis, I was unsure, as was Erin, whether or not he fully understood her situation. She was relieved when he dropped her down to the freshman team and that coach seemed to know just how to play her, realizing early on that what was a "warm-up" for most athletes became the "warm-down" for Erin. The muscle spasms were very much a part of her game and my clue was when her hand became fixed to her side to support the area where the scoliosis was creating more and more of a crease. Throughout the season my orders were to attend the games, but I was prohibited from ever inquiring about how she felt. I respected her wishes and felt fortunate that my part-time job afforded me the opportunity to attend most of her competitions. But as the season drew to a close, I was sure it might be her last playing basketball. Her deterioration was most apparent, and she was simply unable to keep up with the speed required as the sport became increasingly more competitive. It was wearing her out.

We had seen Dr. Goldberg in December, just as the basketball season was getting started. He shared my concerns regarding the increase in her curve as well as her discomfort. She was still wearing the brace the greater part of the day, but was badly in need of a new one since the changes in her body were a challenge to the mold. Developmentally, Erin seemed to be finished growing, so Dr. Goldberg decided to discontinue the bracing. He talked to her at length about the loss of muscle tone especially in her stomach because she had checked out on her physical therapy program. To me her protruding stomach was a reminder that we not only had scoliosis and lordosis, but kyphosis as well. This was made especially obvious by the poor fit of the few outfits that we had managed to purchase for the start of school only three months earlier. For some time, dresses were absolutely out of the question. Even the best tailor could not help us out. It was a pretty discouraging time.

As Dr. Goldberg noted, cosmetic surgery was possible, but there were always risks. He suggested that we give it some thought and see if the scoliosis stabilized itself, which sometimes happens after puberty. We talked about the increase in Erin's limping on the left side and again, he encouraged her to get back on her physical therapy program. Easier said than done.

As the basketball season wound down, Erin continued with her indoor tennis lessons to prepare for tryouts for the high school tennis team. She had perfected a wonderful serve and her stroke was long and graceful. In spite of this, I wondered how she was ever going to summon the energy for another sport. I soon found out that Erin seemed to have her own little reserve which served her very nicely. Not only did she make the team, she ended up playing varsity doubles. Although I had seen her play on our club tennis team for several summers, I had never witnessed this level of expertise. Tennis was definitely her sport. I followed her team to almost every game. She had a wonderful partner and together, they really did a fine job. Her coach was extremely understanding of Erin's back issues since she suffered from back problems herself and could no longer play competitive tennis because of them. All around, it was a very supportive situation.

Erin's increasing scoliosis was most apparent to observers from other teams, and sometimes I would hear them talking among themselves. Some even figured out that I was her mother and would dig a bit for more information. As long as Erin was not within earshot, I didn't mind the inquiries. Almost always they would ask about further surgery. It was a question that had taken up residence in my own mind as well. I could no longer deny the fact that her scoliosis was hard to miss.

The tennis season ended very successfully for Erin and her partner, Amy. Although Erin had thrived on the whole experience, she was exhausted and the thought of having a little breather was pretty exciting. Before I knew it, my year as a special-education teacher was winding down, the boys were home from college, and Erin was in the throes of her first set of high school final exams.

After school ended, Erin took it easy and enjoyed being able to sleep half the day away. Always being an early riser, I was amazed at how much time an adolescent of the '90s spends in a bed. As we got into July, it was clear that one of the reasons Erin spent so much time there was her exhaustion from carrying such a tilted body around. She complained more and more about her back; some of her muscle spasms were pretty severe and they also seemed to last longer. We had seen Dr. Goldberg in the spring and again in the summer. Erin's spine, although severely curved, remained stable. In addition to her scoliosis, she had developed a snapping hip band or tendon slipping over the bones of the hip, which was annoying her more than anything else. She was given some stretching exercises, which helped, but once again, added more time to the regimen she was already doing. The question of surgery continued to surface but, as always, the final decision rested with us.

Dr. Scott had also seen Erin just before her school year ended. She continued to share with him her headache and nausea issues to which he had no particular insight. Her scoliosis was at about 55° at this time, and again he made note of the fact that for such a beautiful young lady, this was a heavy burden to carry. He strongly urged us to go for a second opinion. Being at a distance, he probably had the most objective eye of all, but at the time I didn't see it. The thought of leaving a team that had been so outstanding was hard for me to imagine. In fact, I had become so attached to them as people that I, too, had lost my objectivity. It wasn't a question of competence; it was perspective.

It was clear to me that we were perhaps going down a "dead end." In fact, about six months later, Erin wrote a high school English paper about her back entitled, "A Dead End." Kevin continued to be optimistic about avoiding further surgery, and Erin continued to unload with me how much she hated the way she looked and her increasing discomfort with her body. Along the way, I was beginning to realize that the nausea and headaches were probably emotionally based, as Erin tried so hard to convince herself that she really didn't look that tilted. No longer could she wear stripes or plaids and she was now into boy's jeans because her waist was disappearing. She had become so discouraged that she almost never did her exercises, which only exacerbated her pain as well as her deteriorating appearance.

My dog became my confidant that summer and, as he walked me, I thought back to the very beginning. When Erin's doctors had mentioned the possibilities of regression in all that they had corrected in her very first operation, I must have been on another wavelength. Since this regression or perhaps I should say "progression" came over time, I never really considered that it could get this severe. It was clear to me that still, after all these years and after all my reading, I knew very little about this hand Erin had been dealt. The rules always seemed to be changing.

In August of 1992 we took what we thought might be our last family vacation. The boys were now young men and preferred to travel with college friends, not unlike any of us when we were their age. They knew that Erin missed their company, and so they agreed to do one last fling. Needless to say, Kevin and I felt ecstatic about the fact that they were willing to tolerate the old folks one last time. We headed for Italy, since Breen had an interest in studying there at some point, and we added a quick stopover to explore the south of France. Although we paced the trip in such a way as to accommodate Erin, it was absolutely exhausting for her and many a day we didn't leave the hotel until almost lunchtime. And it was clear that the curiosity factor about her back had become something of a tourist attraction. It was hard for me to tolerate the side comments that I couldn't help overhearing, and I knew that Breen and Colin must have been aware of it as well. At first it made me sad but as the trip continued, it was really making me angry.

The point of reckoning came when Erin and I had stopped at a café in Florence for lunch. We had been there before, but Erin had decided on this particular day that she was in the mood for something different. She got up and walked over to the wall to look at the menu. A family sitting with their two little girls off to my right began a discourse. One of their little girls asked the mother what was wrong with Erin. The other little girl interrupted her sister and asked if it hurt. Then the first asked if it could be fixed. The mother began to explain that some people don't use doctors and, just as she began her next sentence, Erin arrived back at our table. I wanted to go over and set them straight. Erin was also aware of the stares, and I often wondered if she had ever heard such a conversation herself. It's amazing how people need to dissect those with differences.

I carried that little scene in the café with me for a long time and finally made the decision to move on and explore surgery. School had started and Erin was again experiencing the nausea and headaches. My concern was growing, and I wondered what the future would bring if all this continued.

I had no idea where to begin. Dr. Goldberg had told us early on that the operation she needed was not one that he would do himself, and I respected his honesty. Since one of the major concerns was the area around where her diastematomyelia had been located, I decided to get a second opinion from a neurosurgeon whom we knew from a committee Kevin was on. I remember going to the September board meeting with Kevin and cornering this doctor, hoping that he would agree to look at Erin's case. Bless him for being so polite and such a good listener. I explained that her curve seemed to have increased once again, which I had surmised from the way her clothing fit. He requested that we have a complete set of MRIs done and send them on to him in Chicago. Such an inappropriate thing to do to a doctor on his evening out and clearly an indication of how concerned I had become. This was even affecting my social graces!

Dr. Goldberg was wonderful about arranging for the MRIs, and we made sure that we ordered every view possible to avoid any repeat performance. In fact, after they finished, I asked if Erin could look at the images of her back on the computer screen. The doctor was kind enough to give both of us a lesson in anatomy. Erin was fascinated and so appreciative.

A few days later, I went in and picked up copies of the MRIs, sent them off to the neurosurgeon in Chicago, and anxiously awaited his input. Within about a week he called. He agreed that surgery was always a risk for a patient with Erin's history, but he encouraged me to move on.

I approached both Dr. Goldberg and Dr. Scott for suggestions of physicians whom they felt would be able to look at a package like Erin's and perhaps even operate. Early on Dr. Scott had suggested Dr. John Hall, who was also at Children's Hospital in Boston and extremely knowledgeable in the area of congenital scoliosis. Dr. Goldberg gave us two names of people also well-respected in this area: one in California and one in Kansas. Since Dr. Hall was in the Boston area, it seemed appropriate to see him first.

Preparing Erin to see another orthopedic surgeon was not easy, so I made sure we had a bit of lead time before her appointment. She had known for quite a while that if things continued to progress and surgery was likely, it was not an operation that Dr. Goldberg would perform. Nevertheless, they had a special relationship and moving on to someone else, even just for another opinion, was not so easy. Meanwhile, the progression of the curve seemed to continue. Her clothing was my barometer and we were still having to buy bigger sizes to mask what was underneath as well as becoming more and more limited in regard to almost everything she wore. The nausea was becoming the norm rather than the exception, and my concern was growing.

∞∞

The highlight of the fall for Erin was my discovery of a wonderful designer who was willing to make Erin a dress for her semi-formal the following February. I had approached many dressmakers before; I even carried a photo of Erin along with me, and each time they commented on how difficult it would be to fit her. Thank God I had the good sense to leave Erin home, and I never shared any of the feedback with her. When I finally found Sondra Celli, it was only good news, and the fact that Erin could once again have a dress was very exciting. I decided after that, that if I ever won the lottery, I would create a fund so that Sondra was available to other scoliosis patients who might not be able to afford such a luxury.

Sondra first made Erin's dress out of muslin to create a workable pattern. She cleverly designed a dress with two side zippers since a back zipper would not lie straight on Erin's curved body and would only serve as a hint to someone that things were not straight "back" there. The neck of the dress was a cowl style, but Sondra placed elastic around it so that Erin could adjust it in such a way as to have one side up higher, since one shoulder was really slumping at the time. She put a light layer of chiffon over the dress to give a layered look to the bottom so no one could see that one side dipped down lower than the other. To accommodate Erin's protruding hip, Sondra began a subtle A-line to the dress beginning above the hips. The final touch was having a rolled hem so that no one could see the depth or unevenness at the bottom. The fruit of her labor was a dress that was simple but elegant and the burgundy color complemented Erin's blond hair perfectly. Erin's elation was certainly worth all the fittings. By the time we were finished, Sondra and her assistants were like family to us and remain so today.

A few days before Erin's dance it was time to see Dr. Hall. We had an early morning appointment so that Kevin could come along. I had arranged for a set of Erin's MRIs to be sent over prior to our visit. I had the rest of her history in my head, which I had replayed so many times that I knew most of it by heart.

We were first visited by Dr. Hey, Dr. Hall's chief resident, who was both pleasant and understanding of our situation as well as respectful of Erin's degree of modesty. His only comment was in regard to how impressive her curve was. I think what he really meant was "progressive."

Dr. Hey was soon followed by Dr. Hall and an entourage of young physicians who trailed behind. Dr. Hall had that same air of confidence that we had enjoyed with Dr. Goldberg. A man in his late sixties, he had a very gentle way with Erin and carefully guarded his questions as well as his impressions. It was clear to him that the progression of Erin's curve was at a serious stage and was running the risk of affecting her vital organs, especially her pulmonary function. His examination was calculated, thorough, and informative. He encouraged us to make up our minds as soon as possible, for Erin's sake.

We were most appreciative of his time and I explained that we had one more appointment before we could make a decision. As we left Children's and discussed our visit, Kevin seemed to be accepting the fact that Erin might not have a choice in regard to further surgery, and that I hadn't lost my noodle at all. He finally realized that what had been elective surgery just a few months earlier might now be compulsory.

Erin's reaction was somewhat surprising. I expected her to be distressed that surgery might well be the only solution. I was so wrong and I remember the monologue all the way home as she shared all the different times she had fantasized that someone had straightened her out a bit. We did a little reality testing as we discussed that the risk of paralysis was still in the picture. Overall, it was clear to me that Erin absolutely hated the way she looked, not to mention her ongoing back pain.

⌾⌾

At the same time I was pursuing Dr. Hall, I also followed up on a surgeon whom Dr. Goldberg had suggested, Dr. Marc Asher, at the University of Kansas Medical Center. As a member of the Scoliosis Research Society (which Dr. Hall had served as the second president), I knew he would have access to information that might shed some light on Erin's condition.

I must say that getting an appointment with Dr. Asher was like calling heaven and asking God if you could go up and check out the accommodations. Kevin could not believe how determined I had become in my quest. I knew if Dr. Goldberg suggested him, Dr. Asher was certainly worth seeing. I called his office every morning and every afternoon for over a week. Each time they would tell me I had a six-month wait. I knew we couldn't wait that long. Finally, I asked if I could at least send Erin's MRIs, but they didn't want them without Erin. I think I finally got the appointment because I drove them crazy. "He can see you on February 23rd at ten," his administrative assistant replied. "If you can't make that, we'll see you in June."

February 23 happened to fall at the end of our school winter vacation break. Erin and I had gone up to Vermont at the beginning of the week, but at this point skiing was tiring for her and she would poop out after only a few runs. If I could have taken Erin's expertise and form on the slopes and put it in my own body, I would have been quite the skier myself. Since this was not possible, we both packed it in and headed home.

Kansas City is not an easy place to get to by a direct route from Boston. We ending up flying to Washington, D.C., and then on to Kansas. Our first plane had mechanical problems and after about an hour, they flew us back to Washington. This did not set well with Erin since flying was never comfortable for her. Finally, we were on our way.

In addition to seeing Dr. Asher in Kansas City, we were going to visit with my cousin Eileen and her husband and family. Eileen and I had spent many, many summers together in Westport, Connecticut, at the beach. Our mothers were sisters. Over the years we had fallen out of touch, so I was especially excited for her and her family to meet Erin.

At last we landed at the Kansas City airport. Erin was exhausted. It was almost dinnertime and we had been in transit for the better part of the day. We walked over to the cab stand in search of a car to bring us to our hotel. A big man with long, gray hair pulled back in a ponytail got out of an old Cadillac and asked if we wanted a ride. He reminded me of Wild Bill Hickok. There was not another cab in sight and it was clear to me he was looking to make a few bucks, so I agreed to take him up on the lift, settled on a price, and off we went. It was about a forty-minute ride to Kansas City. When he found out I was a special-education teacher, he spent most of the trip telling me about his problem with Attention Deficit Disorder and the fact that his son had it as well. Out of the corner of my eye, I could see Erin chuckling. It certainly was a memorable ride. In retrospect, I realized how trusting I had been and how fortunate we were that he was just a harmless guy trying to make a buck.

After we checked into the hotel, we were joined by my cousin Eileen and her husband, Tom. During dinner, Erin shared how excited and nervous she was about the appointment with Dr. Asher. Overall, she said she was pleased that we had made the decision to seek yet another opinion. Although she spoke very freely, she later shared how hard it was to talk about her back with family she had just met. The whole process was wearing on Erin; she so longed to control this aspect of her life. I had felt that very same frustration when her scoliosis was first diagnosed.

∽∽

The next morning we got up bright and early, or should I say, I got up bright and early. Erin was feeling nauseous and it was clear that she was worried about her visit and the fact that yet another doctor would be examining her. If you let your own mind wander back to your teenage years, just to have a physical for school was overwhelmingly intrusive. Erin finally went off to shower and I ordered room service to speed up our departure. I knew we had to be on time. We hailed a cab and off we went.

In my arms I carried Erin's life history. I had every letter from every appointment with both Dr. Goldberg and Dr. Scott. I also had both sets of her most recent MRIs. Erin thought I looked as if I had brought along my file cabinet.

The medical center was an impressive place, immaculately kept. Everything there looked orderly and the procedure we had to follow to register was organized and quick. Within a few minutes we were shuttled off to Dr. Asher's waiting area. After a brief delay, we were led into a very impressive-looking examining room.

A nurse interviewed us first and I showed her my file of information. She asked Erin a few questions and then explained that Dr. Asher had been asked to do an unexpected operation and would be a bit late. About forty-five minutes later he arrived. But before we actually saw him, we were once again interviewed, this time by his administrative nurse. I soon realized that she was my phone pal, the one who finally had agreed to give me this appointment. She took Erin's file and asked if she could make copies of some of the material. She also took the MRIs and the X rays I had brought and announced that Dr. Asher would be right in.

Dr. Asher was quite interesting. You could tell he was way behind schedule as he apologized for the delay. He asked me to explain what had brought us so far and so, for the third time, I gave my speech. While Erin changed into a gown so that he could examine her, he briefed me on the fact that he had seen her MRIs, but might want Erin to have some additional X rays done that same day. I knew that Erin would not be thrilled, but I also knew that she would do what was needed.

Dr. Asher carried a pocket-sized microphone in his hand and dictated as he spoke to us. I know it's hard to get the full picture without being there, but you'll have to take my word for it when I say that watching him go back and forth between his microphone and Erin was a very new experience for both of us and rather amusing. I applauded the person who transcribed these tapes since the speed with which he spoke made it somewhat hard for me to understand each and every word. Dr. Asher seemed to be aware of this problem. He continually rewound the tape and played it back for us to see if we agreed, in case he had misinterpreted anything. It was an impressive as well as an organized way of getting your paperwork done. He had certainly mastered a "high-speed" voice that was without peer. I looked over and winked at Erin and knew that she also found the whole scene pretty humorous.

Dr. Asher was extremely thorough. He even gave Erin an interview sheet of her own to fill out and went over how she was doing and most important, feeling. He noted that his examination of Erin revealed a right thoracic lordosis with her left shoulder significantly lower than her right, as well as the rotation of her trunk. He also cited that Erin's gait favored walking on the side of her left foot. Within the first forty-five minutes he commented that there was no doubt in his mind that there was a need for surgery and that getting close to the apex of Erin's significant curve and anchoring it would not be easy. He explained that he would go into the procedure in depth after Erin's X rays were taken.

After that it was almost time for lunch. Dr. Asher suggested that Erin go to radiology and then have some lunch. He wanted his own neurosurgeon to take a look at Erin as well. He explained that he would need a few hours to read her file and study all her pictures. As we headed for radiology, I felt confident that we were in excellent hands and that this was certainly worth the long trip. It was also clear to me that this surgery had more risk than I had ever imagined. Dr. Asher had gone into a lot of detail with us and, at times, there was almost too much to process.

While Erin waited for her turn in X ray, I slipped away and called my cousin to tell her we would probably be at the medical center past dinnertime. When I returned, they had already taken Erin. I had never seen so many radiology rooms in my life, and I felt I was intruding as I peered into each one looking for her. Finally, I decided to go to the central station and ask if anyone knew where she was. When I arrived, the staff was gathered around an X ray of a child with a very serious curvature and they were all talking about how incredible it appeared to be. One person asked another the age of the subject. It was at that moment that I realized that I had found Erin. A staff person asked if she could help me. "I'm looking for my daughter, Erin Mahony," I replied. "There she is up there, that's her X ray." "And by the way," I added, "she's sixteen." I must tell you that they were a bit embarrassed, but the whole scene struck me as kind of funny. When Erin asked me how I had found her, I noted that I had seen her X ray and went from there. "You need help, Mom," Erin commented with a grin on her face. We both laughed.

After we were done in radiology, we headed for the cafeteria to eat yet another institutional meal. We used to have these patterns we'd follow after her doctors' visits in Boston. When she was very little, we'd celebrate with an ice cream cone. As the visits seemed to get more complex, we'd head to the second-floor snack bar at the Floating and Erin would order her favorite lunch, fried chicken with french fries. As her condition deteriorated, so did her desire to extend the experience into lunch. But on this particular day, we were both starving. While we sat there eating, Erin was unusually quiet and I wasn't a ball of fire either. Dr. Asher left no stone unturned and the seriousness of Erin's condition came rushing through my mind. I felt that I was back looking at that scary movie I had first seen on March 22, 1979, the day Erin was first diagnosed. All of a sudden, I realized a very familiar voice was paging me; it was Erin asking if I wanted any of her chocolate cake. Neither of us seemed to be in the mood for dessert, so we trashed our tray and headed back up to orthopedics.

When we arrived in Dr. Asher's waiting area, they explained that the neurosurgeon was on his way and would be there shortly. I got the impression that he was not "in-house," which Dr. Asher later confirmed in conversation. Dr. Asher was still wading through the reams of paper in Erin's file, as well as studying her X rays and MRIs.

The only other person in the waiting room was a mother with a little boy who had Down's syndrome. He looked to be about three years old and was having a hard time. She was wonderful with him and seemed to invent things for them to do to make the waiting more tolerable. It was better entertainment than any book could offer, and his giggle sounded like it was coming from deep, deep down in his belly. It reminded me of the days when I used to wait with Erin. Here we were, almost fifteen years later, still waiting.

Finally, the neurosurgeon arrived, and he clearly had already been briefed on our situation. He asked us an extensive number of questions and spent a good deal of time examining Erin's left leg and foot. Erin's level of physical activity impressed him, and he seemed surprised at her endurance and success in sports. He then made a few mental notes, gave her body one last look, and thanked us for our time. Then he left.

A few minutes later, Dr. Asher returned. By this time, the hour hand of the clock was almost on the five, and people outside our room were saying good-bye to one another. Dr. Asher had talked to us for hours or so it seemed. He went over each and every detail of Erin's body and, in that one day, seemed to know Erin as well as someone who had treated her all those years. One of his concerns was Erin's lungs and he suggested that we have a pulmonary function review as soon as possible. He shared with me that many patients in Erin's situation had renal problems as well and so he also wanted some renal studies. After a fairly detailed medical discussion, he looked at Erin and said, "Erin, you are an enigma." He explained that her particular combination of birth defects was the issue and that although there were many orthopedists who could attempt her surgery, he felt that there were only two in the country that he knew of who had a high success rate with this type of procedure. The stakes were high, much higher than anything I had anticipated. Sensing my emotional state, Dr. Asher brought us into his X-ray area for the panoramic view of Erin's life. This was where he had been hanging out all afternoon. As I entered the room I looked to my left and across the whole wall were two long rows of Erin's X rays and MRIs. I could see that Erin was as surprised as I was, anticipating perhaps one or two pictures, but certainly not this many.

From six o'clock until almost eight Dr. Asher went over every single picture with us. As he went through a lengthy discussion about vertebral bodies (the front part of each vertebra) and approaches to this particular procedure, he explained that normally a surgeon would try to stretch or lengthen the spine, but that in Erin's case, it might well be the route to paralysis. He made it a point to tell us that even with his vast surgical experience, he did not feel he could possibly attempt a surgery that demanded such extreme technical ability. The two people whom he felt appropriate to the task were Dr. John Hall at Children's Hospital in Boston and Dr. Robert Winter in Minnesota. Both were recognized in the United States as well as internationally for their ability to do what seemed to be "extraordinary surgeries." I was of the opinion that Dr. Asher was really underselling his own skill and expertise, but he explained that Erin would require a very sophisticated form of motor monitoring which he did not have in Kansas. He made it very clear that this surgery was a one-time performance and that if paralysis resulted, it would be surgically irreversible. He told Erin that she was looking at about ten to twelve hours in the operating room and that the back pain after the surgery would be quite severe. He closed by saying that this was by no means an elective procedure; it had to be done and soon.

Dr. Asher knew that we had already seen Dr. Hall. He understood that although we felt comfortable with Dr. Hall, we had needed to be absolutely sure surgery was the right move and that we had to find the physician who was best suited to perform such a risky operation. Even then, there were no guarantees. Dr. Asher encouraged us to go back to Dr. Hall and schedule Erin's tests and surgery as soon as we got home. Erin said that she wanted to finish out most of her school year, which Dr. Asher felt might well be possible. She asked him a number of other questions as well, all of which he answered with complete honesty. Finally it was time to say good-bye.

Leaving Dr. Asher was not easy and it took all of my control not to let out the tears that were building inside me. He wished us luck and added that we would both need it. His honesty was not at all offensive; it was refreshing and sincere. Never in my life had I ever imagined a doctor spending this amount of time with anyone, especially a walk-in consult. Although today Dr. Asher feels that I would have gotten to the point of surgery without him, I'm not sure that's true. He refers to himself as a "bit player" in all this, but Erin would be the first to say that his presentation of the medical issues clarified many of our questions. It was not hard to understand why Dr. Goldberg recommended him.

For Erin, I think this day must have been absolutely overwhelming and fraught with emotion that she masked extremely well. As we got on the elevator, she commented on what a learning experience the day had been. Each doctor presents information uniquely and for each patient this information is processed differently. For us, Dr. Asher went into great detail, and his explanations helped Erin to understand the parameters of congenital scoliosis. A journey that I had really insisted on Erin taking turned out to be an education in spinal surgery that neither of us ever imagined we might receive. Sometimes a greater understanding of a situation balances out the sadness and one feels more in control. Finally, the decision was really out of our hands and we were sure that the surgery had to be done. This, in itself, was a great relief to Erin.

∽∾

We stayed in Kansas one more day and then headed home. Erin was anxious to get back to her friends and I wanted to get home and figure out where to begin this process. I knew Erin would want to be in school as late into the school year as possible and I was anxious to see if Dr. Hall would be in Boston in June. Also, Dr. Asher suggested that it would be very important for Erin's neurosurgeon to be on hand during the procedure, so

I needed to coordinate the surgery date with Dr. Scott's schedule as well. And finally, I did have a job, and I wanted to try and teach through to the end of the school year if it did not jeopardize Erin's health. For certain, I would be getting my nurse's cap out again.

Erin and I ran the emotional gamut our first few days home. I had a delayed reaction to some of the information Dr. Asher gave us and the potential risk involved was very much on all our minds, especially Erin's. I called Dr. Goldberg, who was very interested in how we were making out, and I also called over to Children's to set up a consult with Dr. Hall. I checked with both Dr. Hall and Dr. Scott to schedule a date for Erin's surgery. We settled on June 24.

Explaining Erin's situation to other people was hard because her package was so complex and, as Dr. Asher had put it, "an enigma." Her particular combination of birth defects were serious in the aggregate, but taken one by one, I got the impression that they were much more manageable. Time was not on our side and had Erin been born fifteen years later, the protocol would have been very different thanks to medical research and state-of-the-art instrumentation. The general public assumed Erin was merely a child with progressive scoliosis. They had no idea what else was wrapped up in that package. The scoliosis was sort of the icing on the cake that came later, but in Erin's case, later started very early and then went later and later and later.

∞ ∞

In the beginning, I was fairly teary, but not in front of Erin. My mind would often wander and focus on what it would be like if Erin's surgery resulted in her being paralyzed. The image was overwhelming. I had gone to see Dr. Hall for a consult to firm up the details of the surgery, but also to feel better about him and our move to Children's Hospital. Although Children's is one of the finest hospitals in the country, it was a big transition for Erin, who had spent some fifteen years in another facility. As Dr. Hall and I spoke, I kept hoping he would see some way to minimize the risks, but he couldn't. He freely admitted that he didn't relish doing any surgery with such high risk and I could easily see that he didn't like Erin's situation any more than I did. I appreciated his honesty and behind all his medical expertise, clearly there lived a kind, confident, and gentle man.

Within a week, I had scheduled Erin's surgery, confirmed that Dr. Scott would also be available, and set up a urodynamics study to check the functioning of her urinary tract and bladder. I also requested the files of her past operations from the Floating so that Dr. Hall would have a complete history. She had experienced some bleeding after several hours of surgery the first time around, so I wanted to make sure everyone had her total picture. No one ever tells you that you have access to all these records and reports; they simply assume that you know. I feel that parents should have copies of everything in their child's file. It's a nuisance to get it all, but it is your child, and you never know when you might need it.

In the ten years that had passed between the last surgery and this, we had yet another medical catastrophe in this world, called AIDS. Both Erin and I had had blood transfusions prior to the discovery of AIDS, but now things were different. Since Erin did tend to bleed unduly during an extensive procedure, she would need to have some extra blood on hand. One option was for her to donate some of her own, which is often recommended. Another source was donations from family and friends with the same blood type. Since Erin's blood type was B-positive and only found in 8 percent of the population, it took a bit of work to find friends and family who could donate. Each blood donor center has its own policy, so it is important to inquire about this within a significant time prior to surgery. I don't think it ever hurts to have a few extra units on hand just to be prepared.

Initially, Erin was uncomfortable letting anyone other than a few close friends know how serious things were or the risk involved. Some days she did beautifully, but then there were others when the wrinkle of worry just sat there on her forehead like a tattoo. She often asked me about the risk involved and even though Dr. Hall had shared that with me, I couldn't possibly tell Erin everything I knew. At times, it was hard for her to sleep and we'd lie on her bed at night and talk until I couldn't keep my eyes open any longer. Even after I went to bed, I'd still hear her in her room. She had her own supply of holy oil and holy water as well as a magic stone for healing. Even though she was private about their significance, I knew that they had their own place in all this. I also knew she was very scared.

Physically, Erin was getting more and more uncomfortable. Actually, she started sharing that she had been getting sharp pains on and off for much longer than she wanted to admit and that she often couldn't get her body comfortable, especially in bed. Little by little, she was letting her guard down and telling me what it was really like to be tilted and rotated. Kids like Erin tolerate pain so well that the rest of us are often fooled by this very tolerance. Just looking at her was a clue that perhaps life was not so comfortable.

For me, the more Erin shared, the heavier my heart became for this beautiful young lady who had done such a wonderful job of making us feel that being "crooked" is no big deal. I think I was probably the only person with whom Erin had ever shared the truth. To go such a long distance, to live such a braced life only to find that the curvature is worse than ever, is a pretty discouraging thing for anyone to accept. Unfortunately, with scoliosis it's often the norm, rather than the exception. In spite of it all, Erin had done just about anything she wanted to do and, above all, she did it well. The richness of her experiences is what made it tolerable.

The urodynamics studies were both intrusive and uncomfortable for Erin, but it was important for her team to know if she had developed any bladder damage along the way. Most important, it would give them something to compare against if there were any complications during her surgery. As long as I held her hand and did a little coaching, she was able to withstand the discomfort. More than anything, I served as a distraction. The people doing the procedure were fabulous and totally upfront in regard to each step of the process. Thank God the results of the test were satisfactory. So off we went with Erin sporting a computer printout of how her bladder muscles functioned.

⌾

A few weeks later we were back at Children's for further X rays as well as a CT scan to see how Erin's vertebrae looked. At that point in her life, Erin had had so many X rays that I used to say that if I put her in a closet she'd probably glow in the dark. As we left the hospital that day, we also stopped at the blood bank to make arrangements for Erin to be her own donor and also for some of our friends to give. It was a full day indeed.

In the midst of all this, Erin returned to the tennis team, playing varsity doubles once again. I knew in the back of her mind was the lingering concern that she might not be able to play again after the surgery if any complications resulted. It was a sport she excelled at and looked forward to daily. Her coach was fabulous and extremely understanding and supportive. Both of us could see Erin's fatigue surface early on in the matches, but we had strict orders to keep still. After the competitions ended she would crash and check out, sometimes for quite a while. Then she'd wake up, eat dinner, and do her homework until the most ungodly hours. But being able to play was important to Erin, and I didn't blame her one bit.

Dr. Hall had also requested a bone density study to check the strength of her bones, but Erin's CT scan results were not so great and he felt that the bone density study was a moot point. Erin's vertebral bodies (the front portions of the vertebrae) were not thick enough to allow entrance to her body from a different angle and so he was left with a more complicated challenge. He would do an anterior approach first, take out a bit of Erin's diaphragm, and work on releasing her past fusions. Then he would turn her over and do the posterior approach. He needed to do a significant amount of fusing as well as realigning her entire trunk. Two bent titanium rods would be placed in Erin's spine with the hope that they could successfully take the pressure off and raise her drooping shoulder. For Erin, correcting her shoulder and the lordosis were at the top of her wish list. The muscle spasms that were coming from that shoulder were significant and made her days more and more uncomfortable.

Aware of our concern, Dr. Hall arranged to see us in early May to share with Kevin and me and especially with Erin what he had decided as an approach. By this time, Erin had also had some pulmonary studies done and it was clear that her breathing was being affected by all this as well.

Dr. Hall was very generous with his time that afternoon. Erin was feeling pretty nauseous; in fact, she was lying down on the couch in his waiting area when he came out to get us. This was pretty heavy stuff for any sixteen-year-old to deal with. The fact that we were getting closer to the surgery date only exacerbated the issues.

It was clear to all of us that day that Dr. Hall had spent a significant amount of time studying Erin's past history and deciding on the best technique for her surgery. He explained that his preference would have been to enter from the back first and divide the old graft, removing wedges from it to allow for correction. Then he would place new bone there, which he would be getting out of a jar, rather than make Erin experience a third incision. He would close that wound and then turn Erin over on her side to expose and place instrumentation in the front of her spine. The advantage to this approach would be that all the instrumentation would be in compression, shortening Erin's spine instead of keeping it the same length or slightly lengthening it, which we knew from Dr. Asher would be very risky.

But Erin's CT scan indicated that the vertebral bodies would simply not withstand this approach. Dr. Hall would have to follow a front-to-back approach, which increased the risk and minimized the hope for a significant correction. As he concluded, I watched Erin's face and the ease with which she accepted all this information. Although it was more serious than anything I ever imagined one of our children going through, Erin's interest in her body and in science gave her great confidence in the capabilities of modern medicine and technology.

Kevin asked his usual questions — how long until she could go back to sports and school —as well as some thoughtful medical questions in regard to the procedure. He, too, liked Dr. Hall and in just a few months had come a long way in this whole process. Erin needed to know she had everyone's support. She did.

∞∞

Finishing up the school year with this on the back burner was a challenge. The highlight was Breen's graduation, at the end of May, from Lehigh. We were extremely proud and totally amazed by the fact that he had already finished college. Those four years had gone by like a flash. Fully enjoying the experience, Breen was equally affected by its ending, but probably for different reasons.

Erin went over to Children's weekly, starting about mid-May, to donate her own blood. Since she was petite and not a huge eater, she was given strict orders to eat hearty and build herself up. A great sport, Erin thought the whole process was a breeze, and she would sit and watch her favorite soap opera while she donated. A few times we were sent home because her counts were not high enough. In total, she managed to give three units, which was a good start. She was relieved when it was finally behind her.

June had its highs and lows for all of us. Breen and Colin were very close to Erin and it bothered them that she had to have another operation and such a serious one. I especially worried about Colin because he had never had a fondness for hospitals. The feedback I got from his friends' parents indicated that he was having a hard time with all this. And as for Erin, she had her good days and her bad and a lot of nights with little sleep. She worried about the pain after surgery as well as the amount of time it would take for her to recover. Nobody likes giving up a summer to rehabilitation, most especially an adolescent.

The support that came from Erin's friends was instrumental to the success of this whole process. I remember a girl who was in the room next to us after Erin's surgery. Her mother related to me how ostracized the girl felt because of her scoliosis and how difficult it had been for her to find supportive friends. This was not unlike other complaints I had heard from other parents over the years, not simply in regard to scoliosis, but for a host of other issues. If you allow yourself to become your disability or if you allow it to rule your daily activities, it will certainly consume you. I was so thankful that Erin had been able to lead such a normal life and that when we sensed help was needed, we weren't afraid to reach out and get it. In some cases, you can do it all and there are still no guarantees that your child will be accepted. This can be especially true if they have to go in and out of the hospital frequently or if they lack physical mobility in some way.

129

As for me, June will probably go down as one of my tearier months, some of which I attribute to the joys of menopause. When I sobbed over a story about someone's gerbil dying, it was clear to me that my hormones were a bit out of whack. On the days when I thought I was doing the best, I did the worst. On the other hand, the days that started out the worst often had the best closures. The fact of the matter was, it was not an easy time, especially since I was often up with Erin talking or rubbing out a muscle spasm until the wee hours of the morning. As I look back on those days, it is clear to me that the support I received from the staff in the building where I taught, as well as the confidence of other good friends, made all the difference. Although we had moved over to Children's Hospital, we continued to receive support from everyone at the Floating as well. When I listened to other families talk about how little help they got, I appreciated what we had even more.

CHAPTER FOURTEEN

The Dream

∞

June 23 was our "pre-op" day at Children's Hospital and it was quite impressive. A nurse assigned to us had scrapbooks on different medical conditions. For Erin, she had one on spine surgery. In addition to reviewing each stage in the scrapbook, the nurse gave us a complete information guide on spine surgery as well as one on the inner workings of the hospital and what was available to us as consumers. After a supportive visit with Dr. Hall in his clinic, we were sent up to physical therapy so they could review Erin's pre-surgical condition as a measurement for her post-op status. Then we were shuttled off to 10 North and given a tour of the floor where Erin would be after surgery. This is such an important piece of the whole puzzle for incoming patients. You can alleviate many of their anxieties by being as informative as possible.

Early on June 24 we began our journey over to Children's Hospital. Erin began her day with the dry heaves, an expected case of nerves. This made for a fast departure with towel in hand and a very quiet ride to the hospital. After a quick examination in pre-op by the same nurse we had had the day before, we proceeded en masse up to the surgical floor. We were one of about six families. The candidates came in all shapes and sizes. When we arrived at the holding area outside of the surgical rooms, each family was assigned a space. Erin was in a different location from everybody else, which she sarcastically noted. Thank God for her sense of humor.

Our first visitor was someone from neurology, who was pasting wires on Erin's head to monitor her sensation during the surgery. Erin was not thrilled, since she loved her blond hair and was hoping it might be the one thing on her body that would be spared. Our next visitor was the anesthesiologist who would be administering the medications during the procedure. He wore this outrageous surgical cap representing the country he was rooting for in the World Cup soccer games, which at the time were being held in Boston. He put in one of several IVs. We had met with anesthesiology the day before, and they had explained to Erin what they would be doing. Then Dr. Scott poked his head in since he would be operating on someone in the room next to Erin's. He explained that he would be available to monitor any issues that came up during her surgery. Finally, Dr. Hall arrived. Kevin and I chuckled at how Erin greeted him. This massive smile appeared on her face and it was clear to both Kevin and me that this child was delighted at the prospect of being just a bit straighter and more comfortable. It was also clear that she had a great deal of confidence in Dr. Hall.

As each of these people arrived, I had an ongoing dialogue with them in regard to preparations for any bleeding. Twelve hours of surgery seemed overwhelming to me and I was wondering if Erin's petite body could hang in there that long. I needed to be reassured that if problems ensued, they would get out fast. As obvious as this seems, I needed to hear it from each of them to allay my own concerns.

As they wheeled Erin off, I still remember that wrinkle of worry on her forehead offset by her beautiful smile. She was amazingly in control and I must say, Kevin and I were impressed she did so well. Once she was out of sight, I could feel tears trickling down my cheeks. Dr. Hall stayed behind to make sure we had survived the good-bye. Kevin and I felt like we were standing there with an old friend.

The operating room family waiting area was a real experience. I had sat in one twice before for Erin, once for Breen, and twice for Colin, so I was fully prepared for this experience. A nurse came out every hour and told us exactly what stage of the surgery they were in. By 11:30 they were stitching up her anterior incision and moving on to the posterior cut, the more serious of the two procedures. The nurse even convinced us to go grab a bite to eat. The change of scenery felt good, and I was hungrier than I had realized. During the course of the day we continued to receive news every forty-five minutes to an hour. Whenever the waiting-area nurse came into the room, everybody stopped talking, hoping that information might come their way.

After 3:30 in the afternoon there were no further reports. Some old friends of ours from Michigan who happened to be in town came and sat with us from about three o'clock on. I wasn't sure if Kevin noticed that it was almost five and that it had been over an hour and a half since someone had come to update us. We joked about the fact that everyone else had left and we were the only ones holding down the fort. Finally, I asked the nurse if she could just call in and find out when we would hear something. A few minutes later she returned to say that Dr. Hall would be coming out to see us in about twenty minutes.

For me, that last twenty minutes seemed more like twenty hours, an eternity. I had a funny feeling inside and couldn't help wondering why so much time had elapsed between reports, so I was greatly relieved when Dr. Hall finally appeared to talk with us. For someone who had spent nearly ten hours in surgery, minus perhaps a few short breaks, he looked pretty good. He began by saying that he felt that we would be pleased with the correction and then explained that unfortunately, without much warning, some pretty heavy bleeding had started and so they got out as fast as they could, rather than risk further complications. That explained the lapse in time. Thank God it was over. In fact, Dr. Hall reported to us that the monitors couldn't even pick up the sensation on Erin's left side because of the past neurological damage. He commented on how amazing it was that she had been able to function so well. He also noted that they did more wakeups than expected just to be sure she could still feel her toes. He explained that wakeup tests are done at critical stages of the operation, after the correction has been accomplished. During wakeups the anesthesia may be lightened enough for the patient to respond to simple commands; patients usually have no memory of this. The relief I felt as a parent I could never begin to put into words.

About an hour later we met Dr. Hall and Dr. Hey down in the intensive care unit. Rather than send Erin to recovery, Dr. Hall opted to get her right into intensive care. We were thrilled because it meant that we could see her, if only for a short visit. It was clear to us that Dr. Hall was pretty excited about his craftsmanship. He was anxious for us to see Erin so that he could show us how much better her shoulder looked, as well as the realigning he had done to her spinal column. He explained again that he had hoped for more of a correction but, in fact, it was far too risky once the bleeding began. He estimated Erin's curve to be about 70° plus prior to the surgery and at about 28° to 30° after.

Although, as Dr. Hall put it, Erin probably felt as if she had been dropped off a fast-moving train, she looked pretty good. When she opened her eyes, she kept looking down at her toes whispering to us, "I can move my toes. I can really move my toes." Dr. Hall gently adjusted Erin's hospital gown slightly off her shoulders so that Kevin and I could see the improvement. It was quite something and, although Erin was awake, I think she was almost too drugged to appreciate what we were viewing.

Intensive care rules had changed a great deal over the ten years since Erin's last surgery. If the nurses and doctors were not conducting an exam, we were allowed to stay at her side. Breen and Colin came in as soon as the nurses got her settled. Eventually Kevin went home with the boys and I stayed the night, a good part of which I spent by Erin's side. She woke up several times looking a bit drifty from all the meds. At about eleven, Dr. Hall stopped by. I couldn't believe the man wasn't already at home in bed. It meant a lot to me that he would take the time to come back and as he walked away, Erin looked at me and said, "Mom, he held my hand when they were putting me to sleep and it felt so good." Although it may not have been a big deal to Dr. Hall, I know that for Erin it was the very last thing she remembered before she went to sleep. That's a special memory and he sure scored a lot of extra points.

The next morning Erin felt pain everywhere. She was also having the beginnings of an allergic reaction to the morphine: she itched and kept asking me if I had known that there was going to be so much pain. I was relieved when Dr. Hey arrived to help Erin work through some of these issues.

I had suspected that Erin was really out of it the night before when Dr. Hall had told us how much better she looked. When Dr. Hey came in that next morning, she was much more alert. He leaned over her bed and asked her how it felt to have a 28° to 30° curve and straighter shoulders. The tears of joy began to trickle down her cheeks. It was one of the most moving moments I had ever spent with any of our children. She kept telling me she couldn't believe that she was going to look better, and the tears continued for the better part of that morning. She even got me started. Poor Dr. Hey must have really wondered about us.

It didn't take long for Erin to rise to the occasion so that they could transfer her up to the floors. It wasn't an easy ride, but once she was in her room they gave her another dose of medication and let her sleep. We had been lucky and were given a private room. There was a lounge chair next to Erin's bed that folded out into a cot. In fact, the first several nights I actually spent more time putting the sheets on it than sleeping in it. Once I leaned on the end and landed on the floor. Erin started to laugh, which only increased her pain. She was not having an easy time.

Two or three days after surgery they removed Erin's chest tube, which had been inserted because they collapsed her lungs as part of the surgical procedure. Her reaction to the morphine got worse and finally the "pain team" switched her from morphine to Demorol. Unfortunately, that didn't work well either. From Demorol they went on to Percocet. Another disaster! Finally they found success using methadone and Valium. Since Erin wasn't able to hold any food down and was no longer being fed intravenously, they decided to give her a few more units of blood to build her up. Things were just starting to look up when it was time to take out her methadone IV and switch her onto Tylenol with codeine. And the final straw was a urinary infection that she picked up from having the catheter in so long. Erin spent the next three days in the bathroom. No one can foresee all these things because each case is different and each person reacts differently. The best advice I can give you is to take one day at a time and know that eventually, it will all work out.

Despite the overwhelming pain, Erin looked amazingly well. The nurses were responsible for a good part of her appearance. Each day they'd arrive full of cheer and willing to please. They knew Erin wasn't having an easy time, but they also knew that it couldn't go on forever. There were days that I wondered how much more she could take. When you're a patient in a hospital after such a painful procedure, you think that the pain is never going to end. That was pretty much all Erin talked about in the beginning. In spite of her joy at the results, the pain put somewhat of a damper on the success. One minute she'd be sitting up and looking wonderful, and a few hours later, it would all fall apart. That was true for other spinal patients as well. I would meet the other parents in the halls or in the elevators and each morning we would commiserate over the night before. It takes the body time to heal and we simply needed to be patient. The cards that lined Erin's walls as well as the other forms of thoughtfulness were a terrific diversion from her pain and a reminder that many people cared.

Dr. Hall knew that I was concerned about internal complications after the surgery, which had occurred after her second operation and served as a bad memory for us all. He visited her at least twice a day and in the beginning, even three times. I think he was as relieved as we were when, after almost two weeks in the hospital, it was time for us to go home. Erin's sense of humor had returned and, although the pain was still rather severe, everything else indicated she was ready to leave. There was some concern about her loss of weight, but I was sure that being at home would increase her desire to eat. A bivalved brace had been made a few days earlier and she had seen the physical therapist for all her instructions. Everything seemed to be in order. Erin had been through a lot and finally, we were on the up-side of it all.

⟨∞⟩

Erin and I were both full of emotion that morning. I remembered back to when we left the Floating after her surgery in 1979. I had had this very same feeling. What can you possibly say to someone like Dr. Hall? Just to know that Erin was actually walking out of there was something, considering what the risk had been. I thought back to the day Dr. Hey had come in to say good-bye, since we were there for the July 1 changeover of resident physicians. He told us how concerned Dr. Hall had been about Erin and her condition and how much time he had spent researching her file. These are the things that doctors don't tell their patients, and, yet, we appreciated that Dr. Hey had shared this with us. It was not hard to understand the reputation Dr. Hall had acquired. He was a fabulous surgeon as well as a warm and caring man.

As I pulled away from Children's I knew what Erin was thinking. It was the first time in fifteen years that we had left a hospital without the cloud of another surgery hanging over us. This was a new beginning for her, and I could only imagine how good it must have felt. Actually, I think she was finding it hard to believe. On the way home she talked about no longer having to put up with the stares as well as the whispering in public places as children often asked, "What is wrong with her?" She remarked that, as long as she lived, she would be sensitive to people with differences. She knew only too well what it was like.

Once home, Erin spent most of her time resting in our bed since it was queen-size and allowed her space to stretch out and readjust a body that was still extremely uncomfortable. She continued on the pain medication for about two weeks and, I must say, that first week she knew the moment it was due. I felt like I had a drug addict in my house, and I had to hold firm in terms of the time span between doses. Since we had two phone lines, Erin slept with a portable phone by her bed and called me during the night when she needed her meds or simply someone to talk to. It took several weeks for her to be able to sleep through the night without medication.

The only time Erin could remove her brace was to swim or take a shower. In the pool the gravity of the water served the same purpose as the brace. Little by little she increased her time and since it was one of the hottest summers in years, she didn't have to twist any arms to find one of us to go in with her. For the first month only family swam in our pool, out of concern for viruses, etc. In addition to the swimming, she also did some walking, which helped to get the kinks out. She had her own goals and her own way of measuring her progress.

Sometimes she would take longer than usual to dress after her shower. I would knock on her door to make sure all was well. Finally, one day she shared her secret with me: she was trying on all the stripes and plaids that had rested in the back of her closet. The raising of her shoulder allowed her to venture into a world of fashion that she had pretty much abandoned. It was a very exciting time. We take so much for granted and for most of us, it's so easy to find clothes that fit. With two different-sized feet and her scoliosis, finding clothes and shoes that fit had been the impossible dream for Erin. At times, it would still be a challenge because of her remaining moderate curve, but not at all as limiting as before.

After about three weeks, we went back for our first clinic visit with Dr. Hall. I'm not sure how well the resident who arrived first knew Erin's case. After he saw her back, he looked a bit perplexed as to why we were so excited. I very kindly explained that everything is relative and considering where we started, this was a gift. Just the fact that the screws and the rod would prevent progression of her curve was something, as well as Erin's joy at being two inches taller, which made her five feet one and a half inches. Finally, she had almost straight shoulders. Although the fairy tale would have been great, Erin got the dream and that was pretty special in and of itself. She was straighter and taller, her shoulder was up, and her lordosis was 50 percent better. Most important, Dr. Hall was pleased with how Erin was doing and the fact that, hopefully, this beautiful young lady might live a less painful and straighter life than the past few years had proven to be. Although we knew that the scoliosis would always be a part of Erin, at last it no longer ruled her life. It merely shared it.

CHAPTER FIFTEEN
Looking 'Back'

T he passage of time has almost a magical quality to it when one looks back on an experience that has such a positive outcome. In some ways it puts me in mind of childbirth. Those incredible last few minutes before delivery quickly fade as you look at your beautiful new baby. As our long summer moved into fall, that very same feeling revisited me. September arrived and already a new season was in the air. It was so hard to believe that it was almost three months since Erin's surgery. Our only reminder of how she used to look was a set of slides taken prior to and during her surgery, as well as a photo I had taken of her back as she walked into the water on a beach in St. John. I never told anyone that I had taken it. I hid it in a drawer and took it out after Erin's surgery. The difference was amazing.

I would soon be back teaching and Erin was about to start her junior year of high school. For almost fifteen years the start of school often meant going for an X ray and seeing how things were growing. Although Erin would still need to be photographed every few months, that mark of concern was no longer tattooed on her forehead. I still get teary sometimes when I look at her as she experiences her own thrill of living a straighter life. I catch myself staring at her from time to time out of disbelief. Most of all, I wonder where the time went.

The summer of 1995 was probably the best of Erin's life since she was first diagnosed. She was experiencing the thrill of her first summer behind the wheel of a car — alone. She had gotten her first real job — scooping homemade ice cream at Rancatore's, a local shop, and she was finally braceless for good (we hoped). I can remember her first night of work. With that wonderful sense of humor, she came home very excited, holding her five dollars in tips. I happened to inquire at the time what she was earning per hour. Half giggling she responded, "I don't know!" Clearly, the most important thing for Erin was finally being comfortable enough to work.

On the days when she was not working at Rancatore's, Erin was helping Dr. Hall with a research project. Still very much interested in medicine and about to begin her senior year in high school, Erin got a little better view of what orthopedics is all about. But I must say that Erin was and is closer to it than many of the doctors who treat it.

On July 11, 1995, Erin had her one-year follow-up visit with Dr. Hall. She was thrilled to be assured that all had healed well and she could move on back into sports and resume more activities. I can't remember when either of us left a doctor's office feeling so good.

In early August we went to see Dr. Scott, who had made a significant contribution to the success of Erin's very first operation, performed her second procedure, and planted the seed for this final campaign. After the exam he explained that he really didn't see any need for further visits. He asked that Erin check in with him in a year via the telephone, but that if all was going well she would no longer need to see him. He did add that in very rare cases, surgery can become necessary in adulthood, but hopefully Erin would not be one of those cases. As we said our good-byes and got on the elevator, it was clear to both Erin and me that we were leaving an old friend.

Erin was not completely free of pain. Every once in a while she'd get a little tinge here and there or she would hear a little noise as something benignly adjusted itself. It was so different from before. None of us will ever really appreciate how much these kids worry in private. Everyone remarked on how truly at peace Erin appeared after her surgery; and we thought she handled things pretty well before. Maybe we just weren't looking closely enough, or maybe our own concern got in the way.

One of the highlights of the year for Erin was walking into a store and buying a prom gown off the rack. The look on her face when she came out of the dressing room and said "It fits!" was so special. The saleslady seemed a little confused and I simply looked at her and said, "It's a long story." Indeed it has been long for Erin. For some, the saga goes on and on.

The three aspects of Erin's surgery that changed her life the most significantly were having shoulders that looked fairly even, a curve improved by 50 percent, though still moderate, and no visible lordosis. All of these improvements made her limp much harder to detect. From time to time, someone would ask Erin why she was limping, particularly on those days when she might have been a bit tired. Most of the time Erin gave very little information and simply acknowledged that her foot was fine. A heel-cord operation would give it a boost, but that still remains an option as is her snapping hip band surgery.

One of the things that Dr. Goldberg used to try to get Erin to accept is that exercise is the key. She has made a concerted effort to tone up and get back in shape, using a treadmill, swimming, and walking. As is true for all of us, exercise is work and it takes discipline and time.

∞∞

I continue to talk to a range of parents of children with congenital scoliosis. I connect with them in a variety of ways and most of all, I tell them that there sometimes is a light at the end of the tunnel. It takes a lot of research, a lot of time, and good medical expertise. Although the numbers of victims with this condition are significantly fewer than those with idiopathic scoliosis, they're out there and they need all the support and information that any parent whose child has a chronic illness would want.

As for Drs. Goldberg, Scott, Asher, and Hall, they remain very much in our thoughts as we watch Erin live the life which each of them helped to mold. What more could we have asked?

Still, I am very much aware that even the best doctors cannot always bring about success. Over the years I have also learned that congenital scoliosis has many guises and can embrace a whole range of other problems. Many cases are far more complex than ours and remind all of us of how truly blessed Erin was and continues to be. Although Erin's road was long, it could have been even longer.

For years I have tried to explain to people how different congenital scoliosis is from idiopathic, and still, much of the world lumps them together. They clearly are not the same, but until more literature is written, the world will continue to place them in the same basket. And more important, parents like us will continue to wonder how many faces congenital scoliosis really has.

∞∞

Bunny Gowen, the past president and founder of the National Scoliosis Foundation, who had presented the Belmont School Committee her rationale behind the need for scoliosis screening in the public schools so many years ago, is now a friend. I receive her organization's quarterly newsletter, *The Spinal Connection;* it is one of the only regular resources available to families of children with scoliosis. There is still a dearth of information. That was my one taste of reality as I sought out someone who had written about the experience. There are a handful of other books on the market, but finding them in a bookstore or library is quite a challenge. And, as for me, I continue to give support to other families who are on the same "crooked" path that we once trod.

I've spent every free moment I could weasel out of my days trying to finish this book, knowing that the story of Erin's life is far from done. This volume was my attempt at sharing a bit of how Erin has evolved. It's taken me most of these last seventeen years to put into words my own definition of scoliosis. It is a sneaky disorder that traverses the spine, calculating its progression with a mind all its own. It teases you into thinking that perhaps it has left, when, in fact, it has merely altered its route. It's a stubborn condition and one that causes as much embarrassment as it does pain. It becomes the best friend that you wish you had never met.

For most of the last seventeen years I would look at Erin and wonder to myself, What can I give you? As a parent you watch helplessly as your child's spine twists and bends. You stand in awe of that power and you quietly pray for a miracle. For children like Erin, who have a rather complex package, there are no miracles. But there is the fulfillment of a dream or two. I realize now that over the last seventeen years, Erin has taught me that what is really important is not what I can give to her but what Erin can, could, and continues to give to the world, in spite of her scoliosis. It is a lesson in life that I never would have found in a book, one that I thought I knew until I lived it, and clearly one that I think is worth sharing.

In 1988 the students in Erin's fifth-grade class were asked to write a paper entitled "If I Were President." In many ways this paper best describes what and who Erin is all about.

If I Were President

By Erin Mahony

I f I were the President of the U.S.A. I would try and make it so everyone would have a place to live and have food to eat. Also I would try to make it so poor people have enough money to live.

I would do almost anything I could to help people with cancer, scoliosis, AIDS, and just plain old illnesses. And I would help elders.

I would also make taxes appropriate for their causes. If it was needed I would make it so that there was more care in hospitals. I would make schools better in any way I could. And I would try to and make it so everyone who wanted and needed a job would get one. Also, I'd make it so there were no cities or states that were too crowded. And finally I would do anything I could do that hasn't been done to stop more people from using drugs or smoking.

If you put everything I just said into one sentence you would probably say I would help people in all sorts of different ways.

EPILOGUE

A New Beginning: Off to College

⚭

June 9, 1996, was a bit overcast, but the high school graduation ceremony would be brief, and we hoped the skies would smile down on the Class of 1996. Erin was excited and yet somewhat nostalgic about leaving behind friends that she had been with throughout much of her life. Over the years they carried her books, helped her in and out of many braces, and even developed some skill at physical therapy. When she had to leave the swimming pool and rebrace, they left too, even though it meant returning to the heat of a 90° day. They called her after doctor's visits, complimented her on dresses in spite of her curve, and are, in every way, our great promise for the future. As they filed into the gym with "Pomp and Circumstance" playing in the background, I saw before me a very exceptional group, a class that would be remembered and missed by many.

For me there were a few teary moments leading up to this occasion, emotions that I had also experienced with Breen and Colin. The actual graduation ceremony was wonderful. Seeing Erin become a young adult, about to move on to a new beginning, was a moment that I used to dream about. Now it was finally coming true. If all went well, Erin would be part of the college Class of 2000, which in and of itself was pretty remarkable. Her high school graduation was also our last, and Kevin and I remarked to one another how weird it felt to be all done. Before you know it, you're looking at your life in a photo album.

The summer went by quickly, a time of "cleaning out" both literally and figuratively. One morning I awoke and found a good portion of the contents of Erin's closet on the guest-room bed with big notes attached to each pile. Many of the outfits had been altered for her more tilted days and I could only imagine how happy she was to get rid of them. Her back is still far from perfect and although finding clothes is somewhat easier, it remains a challenge.

Erin thoroughly enjoyed getting ready for college and loved so many of the things that Breen and Colin had ignored. I remember telling the boys they'd need sheets for their rooms and getting blank looks as if to say, "boring." But Erin organized herself right down to the kind of water bottles she wanted for her portable refrigerator. Her thoroughness is not new: she is incredibly organized and well prepared. All those years of bracing taught her how to manage her time as well as her belongings. What amazed me was how relaxed she was as she proceeded.

Erin continued her job at Rancatore's Ice Cream Shop until about ten days before she was to leave for school. She stayed on a little longer as a volunteer research assistant for Dr. Hall and was delighted that she did. On her very last day he arranged for her to observe a congenital scoliosis surgery on a patient who had many of Erin's birth defects: diastematomyelia, hemivertebrae, and a significant curvature. Other than the time that followed her own last surgery, I have never seen Erin come home so animated, so excited, and so at peace with herself. She finally knew what she looked like inside as well as exactly how Dr. Hall had worked. Although Erin's procedure was twice as long and much more complicated, she had seen in four and a half hours what in a lifetime she had tried so hard to understand. Her relationship with Dr. Hall was and is a special one, and she long dreamed of one day seeing him in action. Once again, a dream had come true. My only regret was that I hadn't been given the same opportunity. It seemed to me that what had been such an albatross some sixteen years earlier had somehow managed to come full circle. It is true that sometimes when one door shuts, another one opens. How blessed we were to see that happening for Erin.

As the final week came to a close, I knew in my heart that I would miss Erin more than I could ever put on paper. And, from time to time, she herself expressed her own very normal nervousness. In anticipation of not being near her doctors for the first time in her life, she requested a card with Dr. Hall's beeper number to carry in her wallet as well as a letter about her surgery since her titanium screws and rods could set off airport security sensors. We also had a note drafted by Dr. Hall for the medical staff at her college. I had sent them her surgical records, but surely a cover letter from the surgeon would clarify any questions they might have.

Early on I had spoken to the house physician at the college and made arrangements for a hard mattress and some gym accommodations. Although Erin was a bit disappointed about not participating in the Outward Bound Program for incoming freshmen, she could now accept her limitations. The college physician believed it would be far too rigorous and in mulling it over, Erin agreed that it really wasn't that important. To deal with the migraine headaches that had been diagnosed the spring of her senior year of high school, we arranged for a three-month supply of her medication. Bothered by this encumbrance, Erin had participated in a biofeedback program over the summer and felt that she had made a lot of progress in controlling this condition. All in all, she was just about ready to move on. Kevin and I did not always share her enthusiasm. But we kept our feelings to ourselves and tried to be "closet mourners."

∞∞

I was amazed at how quickly the last few days passed. Suddenly it was August 21 and we were packing the car, hoping that everything would fit. As excited as Erin was to move on, she took a bit of time leaving her bedroom. She commented to me how much she would miss her bed; she had spent considerably more time in it than most kids. For me, the thought of coming home to what would be yet another empty bedroom was mind-boggling.

The car ride was pretty uneventful. Once out of Massachusetts we made our way through a lovely dairy belt, surrounded by beautiful farms and lots of cows. We all had a great laugh as Erin recounted how a cow had chased me up a mountain in Bavaria some ten years earlier. No longer do I think of them as docile farm animals. It was as if the cow had put on running shoes; I barely got away.

As we pulled into the long, winding entrance of Erin's school, all we could see were cars, luggage, and parents. The future freshmen were the ones with their heads twisting and turning to check out their classmates. We left Erin's belongings next to our car in a lower parking area and awaited a truck to bring them up to her dormitory, which was more steps away than I wish to share. Her room was a huge corner triple located on the second floor of a coed dorm. Both her roommates had already arrived and one was there to greet us. The other drifted in while Erin was unpacking.

The college had done an excellent job of matching up the girls. Each of them was the youngest in her family and the only girl. One of them also had a slight case of scoliosis as did her mother, so she was understanding that Erin would not be lifting heavy things. About halfway through the unpacking process, as Erin was growing increasingly quiet, a young man from her high school graduating class dropped in. He was assigned to the same dorm. His timing was perfect.

The witching hour of four came upon us far too quickly, and it was suddenly time to say good-bye. The lump in my throat was like the one I had some sixteen and half years earlier. I gave her one last hug. Ours has been an unusual relationship, one composed of both love and honesty. Erin has that beautiful gift of telling it like it is which has gotten her through the hard times and given us some laughs as well. How I would miss those moments. It was equally hard for Kevin, and I can't remember a time when he looked so sad. A home that was once full of kids and activity would now seem so hollow.

Fortunately, our sadness was rescued by one last errand at the health services office. We wanted to meet Dr. Miller, the physician in charge, who was delightful and pleased to get Dr. Hall's letter. She made a call for us to the accounting office so that we could make the final arrangements for Erin's mattress board. Unfortunately, the office was about to close, so we would have to take care of that chore the next day. We extended our thanks and reluctantly moved on to explore the area that would be Erin's home for the next four years. After a pleasant dinner at a local inn, we settled down for the night at a wonderful bed and breakfast recommended by a Belmont acquaintance. I'm sure we weren't the first couple to arrive at the doorstep looking so low.

The next morning we got up early and returned to campus to arrange for the bed board. Unfortunately, we had to go from the accounting office back to Erin's dorm. I wondered how I could tactfully do this without embarrassing her. The kids were involved in an outdoor activity and I race-walked by, catching Erin's fleeting glance as I moved quickly past her group. The building custodian had to pull Erin away from her group for a moment. I was thrilled to see her one last time, but it was clear that she had made the break and wanted me to "disappear," which I did.

It was time to move on. Kevin and I took a different route home and explored the Adirondacks, Lake Placid, and Middlebury College, where a dear friend of Erin's was enrolled. We then headed over to Killington, Vermont, where we spent the night.

Once back home in Belmont, it didn't take either of us long before we went to Erin's room. For me, having all the children gone would be a major transition; Kevin still traveled a great deal and, for the first time in twenty-five years, I would be alone. Ordering out for dinner wouldn't be half so much fun and I'd probably have to start giving Foolish a late-night snack so that I wouldn't be eating alone. I was on the threshold of a whole new time in my life. There was no doubt in my mind that it would be rich with new experience, but for the moment, I wasn't quite convinced.

As I took one last look around Erin's bedroom I had a flashback of a nightgown her godmother Rose had given her after the second surgery. Emblazoned across the front was the saying, "You've come a long way baby." Thankfully, Erin has. It was a journey that no one anticipated and one that will never really end. There was a time when I wondered whether an independent life would be possible for Erin. Now, I will spend my time working so that it is possible for your child, too.

⚮

It is now the fall of 2000 and we are in a whole new century. Here is a little snapshot of what life is like in the Mahony family today.

After completing his graduate studies at Columbia University in New York, Breen is now an architect with Robert A. M. Stern, Architects.

Colin is currently in his first year at Harvard Business School, studying for a master's degree in business. He remains very interested in the high-tech industry.

Erin graduated summa cum laude from Colgate University and is now working as a research technician at the Dana-Farber Cancer Institute in Boston. She is finishing up her medical school applications with the hope of beginning study in the fall of 2001.

Foolish, our much-loved golden retriever, was put to sleep on April 26 at the age of fourteen years, one month. As I held him in my arms and watched him drift peacefully into a wonderful sleep, I couldn't help but think about the story he would tell, if dogs could write. He now has a place of honor in our living room and people who don't know that he has moved on stop by and ask, "Where's Foolish?" I tell them, "He's in the living room." After they search for a while, I point to the urn that sits gracefully in front of a photograph of the family that loved him so dearly. "Up there," I say, "so that he still has a front-row seat in this movie we call life.'"

⚮

As I was cleaning out some of Erin's reams of stories and reports, I came across one that she had written back in seventh grade when she was still wearing her Milwaukee brace; it is entitled "Does Scoliosis Really Change You?" In her closing chapter this is what Erin had to say:

"What I've said throughout this story I hope goes for you just as much as it does for me. If you have scoliosis or another disease similar to it or even any disease, you're not some weirdo from outer space, you're just another human being whose body is built slightly differently from someone else. Just because you're physically different doesn't mean your personality is any different from anybody else. The only way you can make yourself really and truly different than everybody else is by thinking you are. If you're a smart person you should know you're no different from me and I'm no different from you.

"It took me some time to learn that I wasn't any different from anybody else and I'm still working on it, but I've learned that there's no reason to make yourself miserable. You're just as good as anybody else, probably even better, because you understand people's feelings and that's one of the most important qualities a person can have. I am very thankful to the people who taught me this, because it sure does make a difference!!

"Just remember, God loved you into being born."

To the Parents of Children with Congenital Scoliosis

❦

The most difficult challenge I faced as a first-time author was what to leave in and what to take out. There was so much to share. This volume is my tenth rewrite of a book that I began almost seventeen years ago and although to many it may not be the "perfect ten," to me it best expresses my journey with Erin. Clearly, each member of our family would chronicle this journey in a different way, which is an important point to remember if you are just beginning the process with your child. My time spent over the years with families of hospitalized children has shown me that one of the most difficult aspects of such an experience is the change in dynamics of the family unit. Sometimes it's a wonderful change, but more often it presents challenges, as each family member searches for a way of coping. Family therapists as well as supportive friends, extended family, and physicians are instrumental in easing the way.

Although this book offers a very positive story, there were many times when each one of us experienced overwhelming sadness and frustration. I remember leaving some of Erin's appointments with the picture in my mind of the X ray we had just seen and wondering to myself, what next! If you are a parent of a child with congenital scoliosis, realize that the emotional seesaw that you may be on has been experienced by many of us. You are not alone. The challenges of the current health-care system in this country have only exacerbated the pressures, not to mention the burden of expenses incurred when you have to relocate temporarily for surgery or treatment, expenses which may include meals out of the home, parking, phone bills, and perhaps a treat or two for the patient. Moreover, scoliosis presents many individuals and their families with wardrobe challenges, since additional sizes are needed to accommodate in-brace wear. Self-esteem issues become paramount, but the limitations of therapeutic services on health-insurance plans force many parents to pay out of pocket for a significant number of the visits or forgo this support altogether.

to all of the above, there is that painful sense of aloneness entering this uncharted territory. How well I remember how ve mentally and emotionally processed Erin's final diagnosis. I realize, as I have noted many times in this book, that we were fortunate in not being burdened by financial stresses in addition to the emotional pressures that all families with congenital scoliosis experience. However, if someone asked Erin today what helped her the most as she traveled this long journey, she would say the loving support of her family and friends. This comes from the heart and is something that each of you can provide. As for the rest, it is my hope that the success of this book will provide a fund of additional resources that other families can draw from as they embark on this voyage with their own child. And so, as you begin your journey, let me be your support. I don't ever mind going "back." I can be reached at 1-800-267-6012.

The Gift

∞

E rin has just finished her freshman year at college. A premed major, she hopes to contribute to the field of medicine in some way herself. Still faced with the challenge of dealing with the unannounced visits of back pain that serve as minor encumbrances, Erin is convinced that the greatest challenge was accepting that congenital scoliosis becomes your partner for life. In spite of this, she has learned to celebrate and rejoice in the many "other" gifts that God has given her.

I will close with this one last thought:

THE GIFT

by Gregory A. Denman

If I were to
give to you
a gift, so true,
Then, my friend,
I would give
you to you.
And you too
could celebrate in
the gift of you.
And I, the visions
of the yous you're to become.

From *"When You've Made It Your Own ..."*

ILLUSTRATIONS

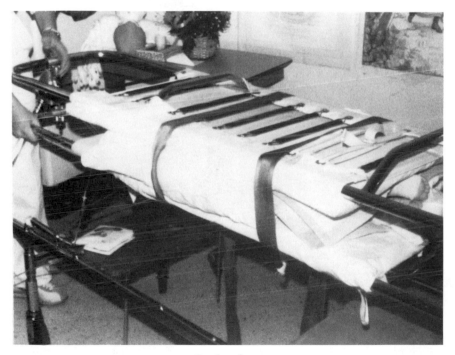

Stryker frame

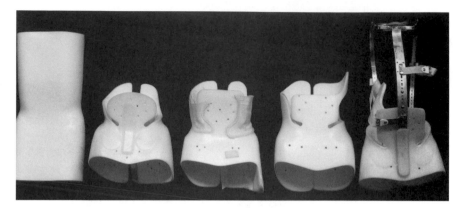

Boston Brace System
From left, prefabricated module known as "the blank"; lumbar brace;
thoraco-lumbar brace; thoracic brace; modified Milwaukee brace

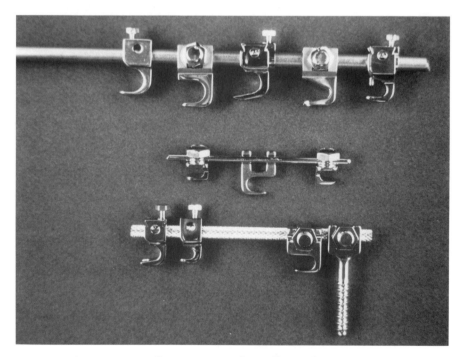

An assortment of various types of metallic implants used in the
correction of spinal deformities.

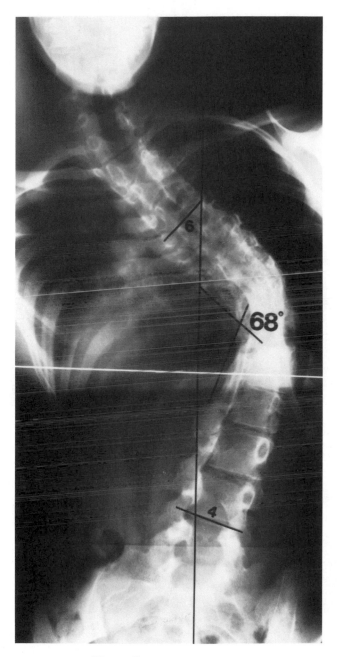

X ray of spine prior to surgery

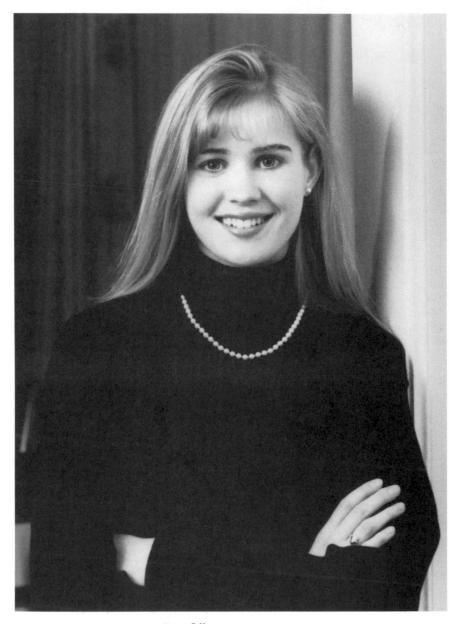

Erin following spine surgery

Origins of Boston Floating Hospital and Children's Hospital, Boston

∽

Floating Hospital for Infants and Children

The history of Boston Floating Hospital can be traced more than one hundred years to July of 1893, when an assistant pastor and social worker named Reverend Rufus B. Tobey from the Berkeley Temple in South Boston was walking on the Dover Street bridge awaiting his train home. While there he noticed a number of women walking back and forth on the bridge, some carrying their infants, others pushing carriages. Reverend Tobey had worked with some of these mothers and it was clear that they were out seeking relief from the deplorable living conditions in their tenements. Accompanying Reverend Tobey was his assistant, Mr. Lewis Freeman, who was along to protect the reverend from what was then a tough area. In an account which Mr. Freeman subsequently wrote, he indicated that many of these women were outdoors because it was recommended by their children's physicians: the quality of the salt air was an improvement for the youngsters, many of whom suffered from a variety of debilitating conditions.

Reverend Tobey and Mr. Freeman soon became preoccupied by this experience and in time, Reverend Tobey nurtured the idea of establishing a hospital ship in Boston similar to one then operating in New York. Not long after the *Boston Herald* newspaper printed an appeal. Donations began to pour in and resulted in the initiation of a formal fund-raising drive.

As a result of these efforts, in the summer of 1894, 1,100 infants and children were transported out into Boston harbor on a barge, where doctors from Harvard Medical School and the Boston Dispensary volunteered their services. Two years later an organization called the Ten Times One Society, which had assumed responsibility for Reverend Tobey's scheme, sponsored cruises that provided treatment for a total of 3,564 children. The essence of the society's philosophy lay in a simple equation:

"If ten workers for good were multiplied by ten every three years, the whole world would accept faith, hope, and love as rules of life at the end of 27 years." The group counted among its members the Reverend Edward Everett Hale, author of "The Man Without a Country."

In September of 1901, the Boston Floating Hospital Corporation was formed and plans undertaken for construction of a large hospital boat to be known as the Boston Floating Hospital for Infants and Children. Five years later, on August 15, 1906, the Floating Hospital made its maiden voyage. The new 100-bed hospital ship was both an inpatient and outpatient facility as well as a site for pediatric research. The most critical issue in pediatric health care at this time was infectious diarrhea, a condition that hit most hard in the summer. The Floating Hospital made important contributions to research and treatment of this scourge: it was on this ship that the first synthetic milk product, now known as Similac, was developed.

Twenty years later the Floating Hospital made its final trip. The ship burned on June 1, 1927, a few weeks after the signing of a fire insurance policy. In time, the directors of the Boston Floating Hospital Corporation joined with Tufts Medical School and the Boston Dispensary, one of this country's oldest civilian health-care institutions, to form the New England Medical Center. In 1931 the new Boston Floating Hospital opened its doors on dry land.

More than a half century since moving to a permanent site, the Boston Floating Hospital now occupies a modern, new facility that provides services far greater in scope than ever envisioned by the hospital's founders. And as co-president of the Friends of Floating Hospital for the last several years, I can attest that the spirit of volunteerism that launched the hospital in the beginning remains a strong force today.

Children's Hospital, Boston

At the time of its founding in 1869, Children's Hospital, a twenty-bed facility at No. 9 Rutland Street in Boston's South End, was one of the few hospitals in the world to care for sick children ages two to twelve. Plans for the establishment of a children's hospital in Boston got under way in 1868 at a meeting of four physicians at the home of Francis Henry Brown, M.D. The subsequent distribution of a pamphlet outlining a children's hospital, in January 1869, led to the establishment of a corporation by the Massachusetts legislature in February 1869. The founders' original document, *A Statement made by Four Physicians In Reference to the Establishment of a Children's Hospital in the City of Boston*, described the object of "the charity" as threefold: the medical and surgical treatment of the diseases of children; the attainment and diffusion of knowledge regarding the diseases of children; and the training of young women in the duties of nurses. According to a contemporaneous newspaper account, the hospital was intended by its founders "for the sick poor of the City of Boston and such only will be received as free patients." Provision was made for those able to pay for treatment and for residents of places other than Boston. In the beginning the majority of patients consisted of Boston's poor, who often lived in unsanitary conditions and poorly ventilated homes, where infection spread rapidly and children easily fell prey to the scourges of the time — smallpox, rheumatic fever, typhoid fever, and tuberculosis.

Prior to the hospital's founding, children were received in small numbers as patients at Massachusetts General Hospital. In 1846 a Children's Infirmary had opened under the leadership of Amos Lawrence and his son, Dr. William Lawrence, but due to widespread prejudices about treating children in public institutions, the Infirmary closed after only eighteen months. The treatment of infants and children was not an established medical specialty at this time. Physicians practicing pediatrics were largely self-taught. There were few textbooks available and no periodical devoted exclusively to children's diseases was published until 1884.

Children's Hospital realized early success and as the needs of its patient population grew, the hospital expanded as well, moving around the corner to larger accommodations on Washington Street in 1870, and in 1882 to a new sixty-bed facility on Huntington Avenue, west of the newly completed Symphony Hall. By 1902 the hospital's annual report cited its continuing growth and stated the need for yet another building to be "erected on less expensive land and in a part of the city where the air is pure and the noise and jar less." Fortunately for Children's, its needs dovetailed with Harvard's plans to relocate its medical school from Boston's Back Bay.

In 1900 a syndicate had been formed to buy and hold a large tract of land for the medical school until it could raise the necessary funds. Twenty gentlemen agreed to contribute to the purchase of just under twenty-six acres of land on what was part of Francis Farm, bounded in part on Huntington and Longwood avenues and Francis and Vila (now Blackfan) streets. Harvard reserved about 500,000 square feet for its medical school; the executors of Peter Bent Brigham purchased more than 400,000 square feet for a hospital; and in 1902 Children's Hospital purchased just under 160,000 square feet. Twelve years and nearly $600,000 later construction on a new 150-bed facility was under way. In 1914 the doors of the new Children's Hospital opened at its permanent address on Longwood Avenue, then a rural, quiet, and uncongested section of Boston.

GLOSSARY

Anesthesia: pharmacologic agents used to put patient to sleep during surgical procedure.

Anesthesiologist: physician who administers anesthesia.

Bone density study: use of X rays to study the strength of bones.

Boston brace: plastic brace used to prevent progression of certain types of scoliosis. Not useful in congenital scoliosis except following surgery.

Bradford frame: rectangular frame of pipe to which is attached a sheet of heavy canvas; used as a bed frame for patients who must remain immobile.

Butterfly vertebrae: malformed vertebrae which resemble the shape of a butterfly on X ray.

Cast: rigid encasement to keep a part of the body immobile.

CT Scan: computerized axial tomography; method of computerized imaging that shows bone detail and gives a 3-D picture of the spine. CT scans are useful in detecting abnormalities and in planning operations on congenital scoliosis.

Congenital: existing at, and usually before, birth; refers to conditions that are present at birth, regardless of causation.

Congenital scoliosis: curvature of the spine present at birth because of abnormality in the shape of the bones of the spine.

Diastematomyelia: a congenital defect in which the spinal cord is split into halves by a bony spicule or fibrous band. This condition must be detected by magnetic resonance imaging (MRI) before operating to prevent problems during surgery.

Dura (mater): literally meaning "hard mother"; the outermost, toughest, and most fibrous of the three membranes covering the spinal cord.

Electrode stimulation: a device for applying electronic pulses or signals for a variety of uses such as activating muscles, identifying nerves, or treating muscular disorders. Electrode stimulation is no longer used in congenital scoliosis having been proven to be ineffective.

Electromyogram: test of electrical activity of the muscles used to monitor muscle problems.

Filum: thread-like filament of connective tissue that can tether the spinal cord to the coccyx causing neurological problems during growth or surgery and now usually detected by use of magnetic resonance imaging (MRI).

Fusion (spinal): use of bone graft to make a solid area on a previously curved spine to prevent progression of or maintain correction to the spinal cord.

Fluoroscopy: radiographic imaging of the tissues and deep structures of the body by means of the fluoroscope.

Gastroenterologist: a physician who specializes in diseases of the digestive tract.

Gastroesophageal reflux: backing up of stomach or duodenum contents into the esophagus.

Heel cord: commonly referred to as the Achilles tendon, which extends from the calf muscle to the heel.

Hemivertebra: a developmental anomaly in which one side of a vertebra fails to develop completely.

Idiopathic scoliosis: spinal curvature which comes on during growth, usually during pre-adolescence or adolescence, and is usually inherited.

Intensive care unit: area of the hospital in which special nursing care is provided for post-operative or seriously ill patients.

IV: Intravenous; within a vein or veins; method used to provide fluids and nutrition to patient temporarily unable to eat or drink.

IVP: radiography of any part of the urinary tract accomplished through injection of a contrast medium; also known as a pyelogram.

Kyphosis: abnormally increased convexity of the spine as viewed from the side; also referred to as humpback or hunchback.

Lordosis: curve in spine in neck and lower back regions as viewed from side; also known as hollow back or saddle back. If deformity is exaggerated, it is known as hyperlordosis.

Milwaukee brace: brace used in treatment of certain forms of scoliosis. Consists of open framework with neck ring.

MRI (magnetic resonance imaging): method of imaging in current use to study the non-bony structures of the spine and other areas. Used in scoliosis to image the spinal cord.

Myelogram: radiographic method used to study the interior of the spinal column and spinal cord. X ray is taken following injection of a contrast medium.

Neurologic: pertaining to the nervous system.

Neurologist: a physician expert in the treatment of disorders of the nervous system.

Neurosurgeon: a physician who specializes in operations on the nervous system.

Orthopedic: literally meaning "straight child." Pertains to the correction of deformities of the musculoskeletal system.

Orthopedist: a physician who specializes in the musculoskeletal system.

Pediatrician: a physician who specializes in children and their development and in treatment of diseases of children.

Physical therapy: use of physical modalities and exercises to treat musculoskeletal problems.

Pulmonary: pertaining to the lungs.

Renal: pertaining to the kidneys.

Rotation: turning of vertebral column around its axis which causes prominences to be seen on the back and is the cause of rib hump.

Scoliosis: side-to-side deformity of the spine.

Snapping hip band: a snap felt on either side of the thigh caused by a tendon slipping over the bony prominences of the hip.

Stryker frame: device formerly used to turn patients without causing movement of individual body parts.

Tethering band: fibrous band which can tether the spinal cord and cause potential problems.

Tomograms: radiographic method of studying bones which permits cross-sectional views.

Unsegmented bar: typical of congenital scoliosis where one side of spine is fused together causing progressive deformity.

Urodynamics: study of function of urinary tract and bladder.

Vertebra: individual bone of the spine.

Vertebral bodies: front portions of the bones of the spine.

X ray: use of rays to study parts of the body.

RESOURCES

SONDRA CELLI
Private Collection

Capable of designing or altering any dream outfit
around any physical limitations.

We love the challenge!

355 Waverly Oaks Road
Waltham. Massachusetts 02154
(781) 647-0589

A special thanks to Anastasia.

RESOURCES

∞

National Scoliosis Foundation, Inc.
Awareness/Action for Early Detection and
Prevention of Spinal Curvature

The National Scoliosis Foundation, Inc., was founded in 1976 to heighten awareness and stimulate action for scoliosis and other spinal deformities. It also serves as a resource center for the public.

The National Scoliosis Foundation:

- *carries on a broad-based, multimedia educational program, working through radio, television, books, newspapers, and magazines to increase national attention to abnormal spinal curvatures.*

- *creates and promotes cooperating networks of educational, health care, and social service professionals from public and private agencies and institutions.*

- *is a resource to persons working for enactment of postural screening acts by state legislatures and departments of education, supplying audiovisuals, pamphlets, and other materials to promote and implement the effectiveness of spinal screening programs. (As of February 1996, twenty-two states require screening in all school systems.)*

- *maintains a resource center of articles, brochures, books, and videos, providing easy-to-understand information on scoliosis to parents, patients, students, school nurses, educators, libraries, hospitals, clinics, doctors, and medical schools.*

- *responds to individuals with progressive scoliosis and kyphosis, as well as to persons concerned about early detection for scoliosis.*

- *has chapters throughout the U.S. offering local support-group meetings and also conducts a variety of educational programs such as spine conferences and postural screening training sessions.*

For additional information, contact
National Scoliosis Foundation
Five Cabot Place, Stoughton, MA 02072
Phone: (800) 673-6922, (781) 341-6333 ■ Fax: (781) 341-8333
E-mail: scoliosis@aol.com ■ www.scoliosis.org